BLOOD SUGAR

Blood Sugar

RACIAL PHARMACOLOGY AND
FOOD JUSTICE IN BLACK AMERICA

Anthony Ryan Hatch

University of Minnesota Press
Minneapolis
London

The University of Minnesota Press gratefully acknowledges financial assistance for the publication of this book from the Dean of the Social Sciences at Wesleyan University.

Portions of the Introduction and chapter 3 were previously published as "Technoscience, Racism, and the Metabolic Syndrome," in *Routledge Science, Technology, and Society Handbook*, ed. Daniel Lee Kleinman and Kelly Moore (New York: Routledge, 2014), 38–55; reprinted with permission of Taylor and Francis Group. Portions of the Conclusion were previously published as "Transformations of Race in Science: Critical Race Theory, Scientific Racism, and the Logic of Colorblindness," *Issues in Race and Society: An Interdisciplinary Global Journal* 2 (2014): 17–41; reprinted with permission of Arawak Publishers.

Published by the University of Minnesota Press
111 Third Avenue South, Suite 290
Minneapolis, MN 55401-2520
http://www.upress.umn.edu

Printed in the United States of America on acid-free paper

The University of Minnesota is an equal-opportunity educator and employer.

21 20 19 18 17 16   10 9 8 7 6 5 4 3 2 1

Library of Congress Cataloging-in-Publication Data
Names: Hatch, Anthony Ryan, author.
Title: Blood sugar : racial pharmacology and food justice in Black America / Anthony Ryan Hatch.
Description: Minneapolis : University of Minnesota Press, [2016] | Includes bibliographical references and index.
Identifiers: LCCN 2015047279 | ISBN 978-0-8166-9617-8 (hc) | ISBN 978-0-8166-9618-5 (pb)
Subjects: | MESH: Healthcare Disparities—ethnology | African Americans | Metabolic Syndrome X—therapy | Metabolic Syndrome X—ethnology | Racism | United States
Classification: LCC RB147 | NLM W 76 AA1 | DDC 616.3/9008996073—dc23
LC record available at http://lccn.loc.gov/2015047279

To all those who live with metabolic health problems
and those who work to heal them

CONTENTS

One month after my sixteenth birthday in 1992, I was diagnosed with insulin-dependent (type 1) diabetes. For myself, and people with all types of diabetes, including type 2 diabetes and other forms of glucose intolerance, a diagnosis of diabetes means lifelong daily self-surveillance of blood sugar and the constant readjustment of treatment regimes, whether those regimes involve injecting synthetic forms of insulin, taking oral glucose-lowering agents, eating healthier foods, or exercising regularly. I often think about my life with diabetes as a kind of war, a conflict I fight on the terrain of my own biology with battlefronts along cellular walls, grocery store aisles, and the pharmacy checkout counter. My particular battle is with a biological marker called blood glucose, or blood sugar. Blood sugar is routinely measured in milligrams of glucose per diluted liter of blood plasma. Blood sugar is a universal biomarker for all forms of glucose metabolism; the ratio tells you how well or how poorly your body is processing the sugar you consume and the sugars that are converted from stored fat deposits in the body. I, like millions of Americans, struggle for survival within these political forces that aim to manipulate, control, and profit from the metabolic processes within my body. I have struggled within the politics of metabolism for twenty-two years as an African American man living with diabetes.

When I was first diagnosed in 1992, the self-surveillance blood sugar monitor I owned took a full two minutes to compute my blood sugar; the monitor I now use takes a lightning-fast five seconds to tell me my ratio. Having checked my own blood sugar on average at least four times a day every day, I have monitored my own blood sugar more than thirty thousand times. If I live to be sixty-five years old, and assuming I continue to have health insurance and therefore subsidized access to blood glucose monitors and the expensive testing strips, I will have checked my blood sugar more than seventy thousand times. Each strip costs about one dollar (retail). The daily self-surveillance of blood sugar can (and should) be supplemented by the periodic assessment of glycated hemoglobin, a laboratory test that provides an estimate of average blood sugar control over a two- to three-month period.[1] I have these tests conducted in my doctor's office at least three times a year, although diabetics can now buy HbA_{1c} testing kits at the pharmacy or the grocery store. Between 1995 and 2011, instead of taking multiple injections of insulin each day to keep my blood sugar within "normal" limits, I wore what is called an insulin infusion device (or insulin pump) that delivers insulin subcutaneously twenty-four hours a day, seven days a week, and more closely mimics the normal functionality of a human pancreas. Pump wearers accomplish this mimicry through increased self-surveillance and increased attention to blood sugar–insulin relationships. Also now available (from the Minimed Corporation and others) are blood glucose monitors and insulin pumps that can "speak to each other" via infrared technology: the blood sugar monitor sends the blood sugar reading over to the pump so that the pump wearer can more easily compute the necessary dosage of insulin.

Despite these advances in blood sugar monitoring technology and diabetes treatment, data from the Behavioral Risk Factor Surveillance Survey (BRFSS) from 2006 show that among people diagnosed with diabetes for whom daily self-monitoring is clinically necessary, 70.9 percent of African Americans, 66 percent of non-Hispanic whites, and 54.6 percent of Hispanic Americans checked their blood sugars on a daily basis.[2] Accumulatively, these surveillance technologies are cost prohibitive, and in the current U.S. health-care system to accomplish diabetes self-regulation really means having access to adequate health insurance and prescription drug coverage. Unfortunately, for far too many Americans—indeed, for many people worldwide—access to basic health care, health insurance, and life-saving medicines is a dream long deferred.

The knowledge of blood sugar made available through biotechnology is life-saving information, especially for people on insulin therapy, or more broadly for people with all forms of diabetes. Paying close attention to my blood sugar and insulin relationships, and thereby engaging in moment-to-moment diabetes complication prevention, has become integrated into an endless cycle that defines my chances for a long, relatively complication-free life with diabetes. Access to these intimate knowledges about my own biological processes necessitates a particular set of social practices that are self-governing, although clearly not only in the negative, domineering sense. Multiple times each day I adjust my insulin regimens according to my blood sugar levels. Over a period of months, I try to use the knowledge of HbA_{1c} to make more fundamental changes to my diabetes self-treatment, such as exercising more and eating healthier foods (low sugar, low fat, low cholesterol, high fiber). By more closely synchronizing insulin requirements to blood sugar values, I can achieve my strategic goal of effective diabetes management. These practices dominate my daily life, but they also instantiate a cycle of positively disciplined regulations that continue to make my life possible.

In addition to blood sugar, millions of Americans struggle to control a host of other biological markers of metabolic processes such as blood pressure, cholesterol, and weight, each of which has its own target of self-surveillance and regulation. I first heard about metabolic syndrome in March 2005. Metabolic syndrome is a statistical construction consisting of abnormal levels of metabolic biomarkers, which, if measured simultaneously in one body (called comorbidity), indicate real risks for the development of life-threatening metabolic health problems. To oversimplify, you have metabolic syndrome if you have high blood pressure, high cholesterol, high blood sugar, and elevated weight at the same time.[3] As a graduate student in sociology, my first research plan was to examine the social and economic factors that contributed to this comorbidity (e.g., having diabetes, heart problems, and being overweight simultaneously) among older African American men. This plan involved conducting a statistical analysis of population-level data that would have, I believed, permitted me to examine the causal pathways through which chronic illnesses developed across this particular population. In the context of this proposed study, I first came across the term "metabolic syndrome" in the biomedical research literature.

A split-image billboard placed in African American neighborhoods on one side shows soul singer Marvin Gaye on the cover of his famous *What's Goin' On?* album, but on the other side shows a bottle of Hennessey cognac with the subtitle "Never Blend In." Sometimes sociology feels like this two-faced advertisement to me: for justice in theory, but undermining justice in practice. In August 2005, I experienced a revelation about inferential statistics, the methodological approach to social research that undergirds large swaths of research in sociology, public health, and indeed across the social, behavioral, and biomedical sciences. This was the analytic method I had chosen for my study of African American men facing risks of life-threating metabolic problems. Through decoupling the subjective experience of people from objective representations of reality, inferential statistics ultimately distorts the already imploded boundary of subject and object. As the harbinger of nomothetic universalism in sociology and other social and natural sciences, statistics consequentially obscures the machinations of social power. The critique of the synergies between bioscience, corporate global capitalism, and state power I offer in this book notwithstanding, I do not want to undercut statistics insofar as I destabilize the very epidemiological evidence needed to document the effects of institutionalized inequalities on people's bodies. The epidemiological work on health inequalities, and the broader bodies of knowledge produced through the use of statistical research methods, do answer important questions about our social world. But they also frame too much scientific inquiry away from questions about the organization of social power, which is what I really wanted to investigate as being important to the health of people living in racially and economically stratified societies. As the result of the research that began with this revelation, *Blood Sugar* seeks to investigate the relationships between knowledge and power that made possible one particular product of inferential statistical analysis, the idea of metabolic syndrome.

Conducting intellectual research as a form of political activism is a defining feature of producing critical social theory, the interdisciplinary body of knowledge and practice that is committed to investigating and contesting the social conditions that produce injustice. This book seeks to establish solidarity with this tradition and other critical scholars of race, technoscience, medicine, and global capitalism who seek to understand the complexities of unjust power relations. *Blood Sugar* represents my own process of awakening from the collective dream of inferential statistics to the unsustainable nightmare of power. I see this power manifested in the embodied reality of and scientific discourses about metabolic syndrome, which both produces and then purports to define the stunning transformations of human metabolism under conditions of modernity. I question the biomedical scientists and clinical practitioners who research metabolic syndrome in an uncritical and apolitical manner, revive naturalist thinking about racial groups, and ultimately obscure our vision about how racism transforms and seeks to profit from bodies. I question the forms of institutionalized racial inequality, modes of biomedicalization and technoscience, and the privatization and scientization of our cultural practices of food and healing that define the transmogrifying kinds of biopower that subject people to the politics of metabolism.

The Metabolic Fetish

In late November 2005, I rode the MARC commuter train from Camden Yards in Baltimore to College Park, Maryland, where I was in graduate school. When I arrived at the station, the 7:20 a.m. express train was just pulling away, so I would have to wait for the 8:15 train. I began to write notes for a critical race theory course paper and tried to enter a reflective space about race and racism in American society and around the world. As I waited for the train, I sipped my hot coffee and ate a small piece of homemade organic banana bread; a few people started to trickle in. An older black man, perhaps in his fifties, dressed in a blue mechanic's uniform sat close to me and pulled out a small Bible. I offered him a sleepy "Good morning."

"How are you?" I asked.

"Blessed," he replied with a smile.

A few younger white people boarded the train, and then a dangerously obese young black man with a University of Maryland bag walked on board. He was at least six feet tall but must have weighed more than 250 pounds. He carried in his hands a twenty-ounce bottle of Sunkist orange soda and two chocolate glazed donuts from the Baltimore convenience store Royal Farms. "This is going to be his breakfast," I thought, and he proceeded to eat both donuts and drink all of the soda before our train arrived in College Park. Although I made the journey to College Park sitting directly behind him on the train and close to him on the campus shuttle from the College Park Metro Station, I never spoke to him, despite my observation that mornings, especially cold ones, can be quiet times on public transportation, although we likely shared frustration with the woman talking loudly on her cell phone who sat across the aisle from us.

If I could have shared my own lived experience with diabetes and my emerging knowledge of metabolic syndrome with this young man, what would I have said? On the other hand, should I even be talking *to him*? Are there other more culpable and influential audiences to whom I should address my concerns? I found myself wondering: Was my silent witness of the young man's metabolic syndrome part of Martin's dream or Malcolm's nightmare? Why was my brother eating this poison for breakfast with a full day ahead of him? Why is it even *possible* for him to buy this food? I certainly suspected that he probably "had" metabolic syndrome even if he hadn't been formally diagnosed with it already. While I had lingering suspicions at the time that this idea of metabolic syndrome was problematic in ways I had yet to discover (as a racist representation of a metabolic crisis in America and around the world), I believed that this young man, and so many of the world's oppressed peoples, was being killed on an installment plan for *nothing less* than profit, privilege, and power.

According to the National Library of Medicine, the central library of the National Institutes of Health (NIH), metabolism encompasses all the physical and chemical processes within the body that create and use energy.[1] While metabolism encompasses a litany of bodily processes that are linked to the development of poor health, a particular cadre of metabolic problems has increasingly assumed a new spotlight in the biomedical research community. Heart disease, type 2 diabetes, obesity, and stroke have all become predominant health problems and are the leading causes of death in contemporary America. An expanding set of descriptions connects these problems of human metabolism to the social and economic conditions of modernity, such as increasing leisure time and more widespread economic prosperity. Some have called these metabolic conditions diseases of comfort because they are increasingly prevalent among the populations of Western nations that enjoy an overabundance of food and leisure.[2] Others have called these conditions diseases of affluence, a label that emphasizes the positive statistical correlations between social class and metabolic illness.[3] This shift from infectious and communicable diseases to chronic metabolic conditions as leading causes of death has been called "the epidemiologic transition."[4]

Although diseases like heart disease and diabetes are now part of Americans' daily conversations, since 1956 biomedical researchers, government agencies, and the pharmaceutical industry have increasingly used a new term, "metabolic syndrome," to describe the observed comorbidity of metabolic states linked to the health risks of heart disease, diabetes, and obesity.[5] Metabolic syndrome is metabolic because it concerns the biological processes by which bodies metabolize nutrients derived from food and describes these processes in terms of physiological or biochemical indicators of disease processes that are measured at the level of an individual's biology and biochemistry. Specifically, metabolic syndrome is a combination of clinical and laboratory measurements that represent the likely development of metabolic health problems: elevated blood pressure, elevated cholesterol, elevated blood sugar, and elevated weight.[6] Metabolic syndrome is a syndrome precisely because it is an aggregation of clinical and laboratory measurements that has not yet reached designation as a disease.[7] Metabolic syndrome represents the collection of measurements of hypertension, dyslipidemia, hyperglycemia, and obesity, each of which biomedical researchers and epidemiologists have identified as major so-called risk factors for heart disease, diabetes, and stroke. According to an analysis of the 1988–94 National Health and Nutrition Examination Survey (NHANES), a nationally representative study of the major adult populations in the United States, nearly one out of four (23.7 percent), more than sixty million people, could potentially be classified with metabolic syndrome.[8]

The fact that high proportions of Americans can be classified with metabolic syndrome has helped to establish a context where a range of biomedical, government, and corporate social actors has taken up metabolic syndrome in their work. For example, in 2000, an iteration of metabolic syndrome (then named dysmetabolic syndrome X) was given a diagnostic code (277.7) in the World Health Organization's International Classification of Disease (ICD-9). In 2002, a group of biomedical researchers started the Metabolic Syndrome Institute, an independent and not-for-profit organization that is the first organization dedicated to the dissemination of knowledge about metabolic syndrome.[9] In 2003, a new academic journal was established to publish research articles specifically on metabolic syndrome and its related disorders. Metabolic syndrome is also the subject of numerous medical books and monographs intended for the lay public, physicians, mental health professionals, and animal and biomedical researchers.[10] The volume of published biomedical research literature on metabolic syndrome is substantial and the rate of new publications has steadily increased in recent years.[11] In 1989, as Figure 1 shows, only one article was published on metabolic syndrome and related terms. By 2012, 4,805 articles were published on metabolic syndrome, representing a 2,000 percent increase in publications over a twenty-year period.

Scientists from across biomedicine, the government, and pharmaceutical corporations use metabolic syndrome as a new way to describe and

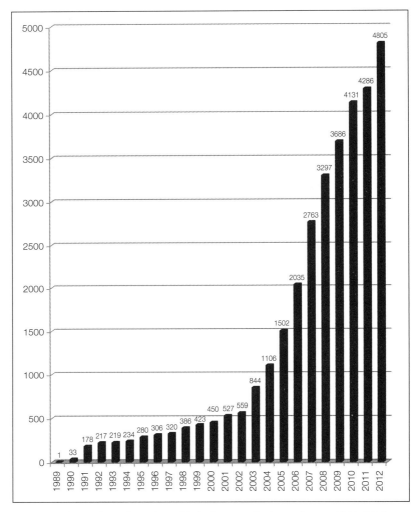

Figure 1. The number of articles published on metabolic syndrome, 1989–2012.

respond to the increasing challenges that multiple metabolic conditions present to Americans' health. Despite the increasing visibility of metabolic syndrome, it would be a mistake to assume that the names, definitions, and meanings of the syndrome have been consistent within this exponentially growing body of biomedical literature. While early iterations of metabolic syndrome were formulated between the 1940s and 1980s, research on it began to accelerate in the 1990s and continued into the new millennium. Using widely accepted statistical techniques such as factor analysis and linear regression, biomedical researchers have correlated metabolic syndrome with an impressive and sobering array of health conditions, including stroke, kidney failure, polycystic ovarian syndrome, cancer, HIV, and erectile dysfunction.[12] These statistical associations are possible because the metabolic states that encompass metabolic syndrome unfold via multiple systems of the biological body. Cardiologists and endocrinologists use the syndrome as a statistical predictor of who is most likely to develop heart disease and type 2 diabetes.[13] Psychiatrists and mental health researchers note the associations between metabolic syndrome and mental disorders such as schizophrenia, bipolar disorder, and depression.[14]

In addition to biomedical researchers, government institutions that conduct biomedical research focused on health and medicine, such as the National Institutes of Health and the Food and Drug Administration, also focus on metabolic syndrome. In 2001, the National Cholesterol Education Program (NCEP) of the National Heart, Lung, and Blood Institute (NHLBI), part of the National Institutes of Health, defined metabolic syndrome as a potential target of biomedical intervention in its landmark guidelines on how to address the problem of high cholesterol among Americans.[15] The federal government also coordinates clinical trials for prescription drugs that might be associated with metabolic syndrome. In October 2013, a search of the clinicaltrials.gov Web site that solicits research subjects for federally regulated clinical trials found 1,092 projects that list metabolic syndrome as a condition under study.[16] Twenty-one percent of these studies (228 studies) are funded by the pharmaceutical industry; the federal government agencies, including the NIH, sponsor 169 studies; the remaining 695 are sponsored by individuals, universities, and other organizations. Figure 2 shows the locations of these studies; the vast majority of these open studies recruit participants in the United States and Europe.

Ninety percent of the global market for prescription drugs is in the United States, Europe, and Japan. Given deepening global economic problems, patented prescription drug sales are at thirty-year lows (adjusted for inflation) because of the increasing market share of generic medications, slower Food and Drug Administration (FDA) approval processes, and fewer blockbuster drugs.[17] In this context, pharmaceutical corporations are interested in developing prescription drugs that could be sold to people who might be classified with metabolic syndrome. Indeed, the health problems encapsulated by metabolic syndrome currently account

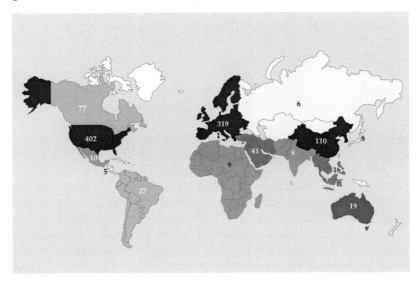

Figure 2. The number of active clinical trials recruiting for metabolic syndrome, 2013.

for one-fifth of health-care spending in the United States and much of that money is spent on prescription drugs. In 2012, Americans spent $335.8 billion on prescription drugs, five times more than they spent in 1990.[18] As of 2012, six of the top twenty best-selling drugs manage high blood pressure, high cholesterol, or high blood sugar, three core components of metabolic syndrome.[19] For example, Lipitor and Plavix, which manage risk for heart attacks and stroke, are the two best-selling prescription drugs of all time, bringing in $13.696 billion and $9.927 billion in sales, respectively. Any prescription drugs that treat hypertension, dyslipidemia, hyperglycemia, and obesity are all potentially useful in treating patients who might be classified with metabolic syndrome.

Defining the Politics of Metabolism

Collectively, these increases in biomedical, government, and pharmaceutical attention on metabolic syndrome reflect a growing apparatus of scientific, government, and corporate actors and institutions that are deeply invested in studying, regulating, and profiting from problems associated with metabolism.[20] An apparatus forms as a strategic response to a specific scientific discovery, political crisis, or economic opportunity. In this context, metabolic syndrome is a new discourse in the apparatus that I call the politics of metabolism and define as the ideas, social practices, and institutional relationships that govern the metabolic health of individuals and groups. These relationships operate on several different levels of analysis. At the macro level, big social institutions such as government health-research institutions, pharmaceutical corporations, and professional medical associations represent the three groups of social actors who produce discourses of metabolic syndrome. At the micro level, these discourses, technologies, and practices operate at the levels of biochemicals, DNA, and prescription drugs.

Understanding metabolic syndrome requires that we shift our thinking from an *epidemic* perspective to one that embraces an *endemic* view of metabolic health problems. Recent scientific discourse about the metabolic problems that comprise metabolic syndrome refers to each of them as epidemics in their own right.[21] Epidemics are viral or bacterial infections from outside the body that quickly and indiscriminately kill large numbers of individuals living within a circumscribed geographic location. While it is true that most Americans will most likely experience and/or die from one or more metabolic problems, these conditions are not epidemics in the historical sense of the term. The historical response to controlling and eradicating epidemics has been to rapidly target individuals who are most likely to fall within the epidemic's relational and spatial reach.

In stark contrast, the politics of metabolism is characterized by endemic problems. Endemics are discriminating, widespread, and long-term population-level phenomena that weaken societies' energies because treating them is expensive and they lead to the decreased economic productivity of working populations.[22] According to data published by leading authorities, the direct and indirect health-care costs from heart disease, diabetes, and stroke exceed one trillion dollars per year.[23] Because endemics represent a political problem for those who govern, endemic problems quickly become objects of government intervention, scientific disciplines, and capitalist expansion. In the context of improved health and productivity, this framing of endemic phenomenon is required to excise as much political utility, scientific discipline, and economic profit as possible.

Shifting our perspective from an epidemic to an endemic view is critical for understanding how the biological realities, political rationalities, and economic opportunities of the politics of metabolism shaped the discourses of metabolic syndrome. Developing a more robust understanding of the politics of metabolism also involves analysis of the biomedical-government-industry collaborations that lie at the center of biomedical knowledge production in the United States. Although metabolic syndrome may not exist as a biological reality in precisely the same ways that cancers exist, it emerged in the context of a massive biomedical, government, and corporate response to the endemic problems of metabolism. The discourses, technologies, and practices of these social institutions are the tools with which researchers construct metabolic syndrome. Taken together, these preliminary interpretations underscore both the importance of ideas and institutional practices in the politics of metabolism.

Race, Ethnicity, and Metabolic Syndrome

Metabolic syndrome not only constitutes a new way of constructing, studying, and treating human metabolism, it also serves as an emerging cultural location for the construction of new meanings of race and ethnicity. To understand the relationships between metabolic syndrome, race, and ethnicity, and to analyze the meanings produced through the science of metabolic syndrome, *Blood Sugar* interrogates the uses of racial and ethnic categories in metabolic syndrome research. The first set of relationships that link metabolic syndrome to race concerns the specific constructions of race and ethnicity that are used in this research. Race and ethnicity are socially constructed systems of categorization that are used to identify, group, and rank human beings, albeit based on different criteria. Race is a socially constructed category that emerged in the 1600s to classify individuals into so-called races based on presumed biological differences between population groups. Ethnicity is a socially constructed category that emerged in the 1920s to classify individuals into so-called ethnic groups based on presumed differences in culture, geographic origin, and ancestry. Race and ethnicity are related in that ethnicity emerged in large part in response to critiques of biological notions of race. Given this historical relationship, race and ethnicity are not interchangeable systems of categorization. However, there is meaningful overlap between what are considered racial and ethnic groups. For example, African Americans are considered to be both a racial and an ethnic group. Race and ethnicity are controversial systems of categorization, especially in the context of biomedical research, because individual biological and genetic differences do not fall neatly along racial and ethnic lines. In other words, despite their shared origins in response to biological interpretations of individual and group differences, race and ethnicity are social constructions.

The federal government plays several important roles in the production of metabolic syndrome and race. It enforces the racial categorizations used in biomedical research on metabolic syndrome, funds and produces research on the syndrome, and regulates the labeling and safety of prescription drugs related to it. Because of historical and current federal research policies that regulate demographic data collection, statistical information about a research subject's race and ethnicity is routinely collected along with anthropomorphic, molecular, and genetic information about the subject's metabolism.[24] Therefore, the sampling frames, analytic strategies, and research findings of metabolic syndrome research studies are often framed using these racial and ethnic categories. In this regulated scientific environment, it is also common to see published review articles on metabolic syndrome that are focused exclusively on particular racial and ethnic minority groups.[25] The racial categories used in federally regulated health research are statutorily based on the Office of Management and Budget's 1997 Standards for Maintaining, Collecting, and Presenting Federal Data on Race and Ethnicity.[26] The OMB recommendations on the measurement of race and ethnicity in the general population note that "the [racial] categories that were developed represent a social-political construct designed to be used in the collection of data on the race and ethnicity of major broad population groups in this country, and are not anthropologically or scientifically based."[27] In this context, many researchers also frame their research on racial groups as ethnic to avoid talking explicitly about race in ways that could be interpreted as racial bias, or worse, scientific racism.

A second set of relationships that link metabolic syndrome to race and ethnicity concerns the effort to study, prescribe, and label drugs that may be related to metabolic syndrome.[28] Drug companies are actively recruiting individuals who seemingly have metabolic syndrome for their clinical research. For example, the African American Rosuvastatin Investigation and Efficacy Study (or ARIES Study) investigated the ability of Crestor, a powerful new member of the statin class, to lower both blood pressure *and* cholesterol in a self-identified African American population.[29] A second recent study, the Clinical Utility of Caduet in Simultaneously Achieving Blood Pressure and Lipid Endpoints in a Specific Patient Population (or CAPABLE Study) investigated whether Caduet, a combination of two drugs, Lipitor and Norvasc, was effective at lowering African Americans' blood pressure and cholesterol.[30] Both of these prescription drug studies were conducted in a manner similar to the way that African Americans were targeted in the research and marketing of BiDil, an antihypertensive medication that is the first drug approved by the FDA for use in a specific so-called ethnic group: African Americans.[31] Yet, coupled with recent research findings that suggest that members of racially and ethnically categorized groups might require different medications, dosages, and routes of administration of prescription drugs trials and because of new federal guidelines about the inclusion of racial and ethnic minorities in clinical trials, this research has a new racial dimension.[32]

Metabolic syndrome has become a new way of representing and explaining racial health inequalities in America. The scope and impact of chronic metabolic conditions have intensified in the United States, especially among racial and ethnic minority groups. Recent data from the Centers for Disease Control and Prevention (CDC) document substantial and persistent racial disparities in the distribution of and complications from these major chronic metabolic conditions.[33] For decades, social epidemiologists have documented such disparities among racial and ethnic minority groups.[34] This research on racial health disparities reveals that African Americans and other racially categorized minority groups experience higher rates of death owing to chronic metabolic diseases and higher rates of complications from those diseases, in large part because of the interactive dynamics of racism, sexism, and class inequality on health.[35]

This body of literature on racial health disparities has received less attention in terms of making a theoretical contribution to critical race theory, science and technology studies, or political sociology, and instead has been more embraced in the fields of social epidemiology and public health. At its core, this research challenges the notion that racial health disparities are caused by natural and cultural differences between racially categorized groups. These scholars have long argued that racial health disparities result from group-based inequalities in access to the economic and political resources necessary to maintain and improve health, such as having access to affordable and adequate medical care. However, simply paying more attention to racially encoded health disparities in the context of metabolic syndrome will not be enough. Currently, scientific comparisons of racially categorized groups in metabolic syndrome and its correlates have become a veritable cottage industry. Nobly, metabolic syndrome analysts often carry out their work with the purpose of devising better biomedical explanations for health disparities in heart disease, diabetes, and stroke. Yet, the dubious theories of racial inequality and discourses of race that emerge from metabolic syndrome research on racial and ethnic groups have not been adequately addressed in that research.

Through these practices, metabolic syndrome has become a new discursive tool used to produce new meanings of race in the politics of metabolism. Specifically, metabolic syndrome draws upon and extends knowledge-making practices that have long constructed race as natural, biological, and genetic. As the biomedical discourses and practices of metabolic syndrome continue to unfold, they intersect with the ways in which race shapes the theories and practices of medicine in terms of disease surveillance, diagnosis, and treatment. Because metabolic syndrome emerged largely from within twentieth-century American biomedicine, it was inexorably shaped by the social structures of race and racism. The sociological relationships between metabolic syndrome and race in the United States seem to have emerged at the intersection of scientific racism—a set of scientific discourses and practices that served to ignore, explain away, and/or justify racial inequalities—and the practices of an increasingly biological and technological approach to the study of human metabolism.

Blood Sugar explores how metabolic syndrome and race operate together as forms of power and knowledge within the politics of metabolism. Three questions guide the arguments I make. First, how did metabolic syndrome emerge as a new discourse in the politics of metabolism? Second, how are current conceptions and meanings of race constructed through the science of metabolic syndrome? Third, what are the implications of this emerging relationship between metabolic syndrome and race for understanding the construction of racial meanings and the reproduction of racism within the politics of metabolism?

Genealogy, Discourse, and Power

Understanding the politics of metabolism requires a methodological framework that can analyze the relationships between power and knowledge, which I believe lies at the heart of my questions about metabolic syndrome and race. The overarching theoretical challenge of understanding the linkages between metabolic syndrome and race is grasping how they operate in what Foucault called a polyvalent manner. Foucault used the term "polyvalence" to describe how discourses can be used as both a technique and an outcome of power.[36] For example, laws simultaneously are produced by and constitute state power. In other words, discourse is not only the documented effect of power relations, as in the case of the legal discourse that is produced by the state (discourse as an outcome of power), it can also be used to mark its own material effects on bodies themselves by virtue of an existing set of power relations (discourse as a technique of power). Understood in this context of polyvalence, discourses establish the scientific knowledges that are used to justify unequal power relationships. In turn, these relationships structure the production and content of scientific knowledge.

Genealogy is a necessary methodological intervention to conducting a standard quantitative analysis of racial health inequalities and metabolic syndrome that aims to produce scientific truths about metabolic syndrome and race. In contrast, a genealogical account of the relationships between metabolic syndrome and race would not assume, nor does it seek to posit, any scientific hypotheses about metabolic syndrome and race. Rather, a genealogical account examines the social structures of power and knowledge that make it possible epistemologically for biomedical scientists to produce scientific claims about metabolic syndrome and race.

Blood Sugar is a genealogy of metabolic syndrome and race in the United States. I ground my articulation of genealogy based on what Michel Foucault wrote in his books, essays, and lectures, as well as the secondary interpretations of key Foucauldian scholars.[37] Any reasonable interpretation of genealogy is complicated by the fact that Foucault never codified how he believed genealogies ought to be carried out, and when he did state his method in recognizable terms, these definitions shifted over time. Indeed, he was not forthcoming with a codified checklist of procedures a researcher might follow to conduct a genealogy, and since his death, his interpreters have continued to struggle to do so.[38] Despite the spirited debates about Foucault's codification of a genealogical method, and disagreement about how these methods ought to be deployed, this book offers a grounded interpretation of what genealogy entails.

Genealogy is a historical methodology that traces the emergence and descent of technologies and practices used to produce discourses about the body and the political contexts through which these elements are constructed as self-evident, natural, and universal. Genealogy is also a form of political critique that diagnoses how such discourses, practices, and technologies are embedded in and rationalize unequal power arrangements. The intellectual and political intent of genealogy, therefore, is to contest discourses that are used to instantiate, enable, and support repressive and/or productive forms of modern social power by showing how those discourses have determined (in a limited way) what constitutes our present understanding of ourselves, our social world, and the social relationships therein. It is in this sense that Foucault and others have referred to genealogy as a "history of the present." Two intertwined analyses comprise genealogy, namely, the analyses of descent and emergence.

The Analyses of Descent and Emergence

The analysis of descent documents the heterogeneous sites of knowledge production by tracing the actual research techniques and procedures used in scientific practice.[39] It shows how these techniques and procedures structure what kinds of scientific practices are acceptable and how social arrangements shape the production of scientific knowledge. In this

Foucauldian sense, practices can be defined as "places where what is said and what is done, rules imposed and reasons given, the planned and the taken-for-granted meet and interconnect."[40] Thus, the analysis of descent narrates actual historical events where the objects of genealogical analysis are inscribed by particular constellations of discourses, techniques, and practices.

However, in contrast to a more conventional form of historiography that might produce a linear and modern history of these technologies and practices, the analysis of descent highlights what I call the disjunctures that are central to the inscription of power/knowledge relationships. A disjuncture is an accident, error, shift, or deviation that challenges the assumption that historical events are homogeneous and represent self-evident truths. Disjunctures represent moments where the structure of discursive possibilities either opens up or contracts depending on the particular configuration of the field of power and knowledge in play in that moment. Foucault's approach to analyzing the disjunctures of modern history is directly linked to one of the central epistemological aims of genealogy; namely, to challenge self-evident discourses and practices that justify unequal social arrangements. Foucault worked to carry out this aim without resorting to presentism, which Mitchell Dean defines as "the unwitting projection of a structure of interpretation that arises from the historian's own experience or context onto aspects of the past under study."[41] Based on this understanding, I use the construct of disjunctures to work against the notion that this study is a modern history of ideas and to highlight the multiple open-ended processes that undergird the production of metabolic syndrome and race as taken-for-granted truths.

In conjunction with the analysis of descent, the analysis of emergence situates the emergence of a practice or discourse within a broader network of institutionally based power and knowledge relationships.[42] What is distinctive is that the analysis of emergence should avoid describing the causes, motives, or perceived intent of a given social practice as self-evident, natural, and universal. To the contrary, practices can emerge in multiple sites of power, can take radically different forms in different historical moments, and do not result from one unitary cause. Foucault's treatment of the body illustrates these dual concepts of descent and emergence. For instance, in *The Birth of the Clinic*, Foucault argued that the surveillance of the body was historically organized via a clinical gaze, a way of seeing and knowing the body and nature, that sought to rationalize the space-time between life and death by classifying and organizing the body scientifically.[43] Foucault argued that genealogies should make an ascending analysis of power that traces the descent and emergence of the technologies used in the scientific study of the body and the social regulations of institutional power.[44] In this way, the analysis of descent should reveal how the body itself becomes inscribed through the production of discourses that are produced in service of power arrangements. In other words, Foucault believed that the body was the canvas on which power paints history. Taken together, these components of genealogy examine the polyvalent ways in which the body, the spaces around it, and the materials inside of it became both the object of knowledge and subject to new forms of social power.

Drawing on this notion of genealogy as a form of social historiography and political critique, I also rely heavily on the tools of discourse analysis as a method for the analysis of documents.[45] Rather than only analyzing the meaning of a discourse, discourse analysis also analyzes the structure of the themes by which a particular discourse is produced. Specifically, it asks three core questions about the production of discourses: (1) Who produced the discourses and with what resources? (2) Under what political, economic, and historical conditions were the discourses produced? and (3) How are the meanings of the discourse shaped by these economic, political, and historical conditions? Thus, my discourse analysis aims to interpret how the discourse of metabolic syndrome emerged in ways that draw on constructions of race in service of producing new meanings of race.

The methods of genealogy and discourse analysis bring into focus the types of documentary evidence required to analyze the relationships between race and metabolic syndrome. Each of these documents contains specific information about the discourses, techniques, and practices used in the scientific study of the body. This study analyzes three types of documents: (a) published research, commentaries, and editorials on metabolic syndrome and race in professional and academic biomedical journals; (b) corporate documents from pharmaceutical companies, including yearly reports, regulatory submissions to the FDA, and clinical trial documentation; and (c) government documents, including NIH and FDA regulatory guidelines on the collection of data on race and ethnicity in U.S. biomedical research and clinical trials, published reports and scientific documents from the NIH and its institutes, and other relevant government agencies.

Mapping Metabolism: A Brief Overview

In the next chapter, "Race, Biomedicine, and Health Injustice," I discuss the three theoretical frameworks that guide the book's main arguments (critical race theory, biomedicalization, and biopower) in order to contextualize and explain the relationship between metabolic syndrome and race. I draw attention to the complementary yet contrasting accounts of social processes, institutional relationships, and ways of constructing racial meaning that these frameworks provide for understanding the politics of metabolism. First, by drawing on a critical race framework, I argue that metabolic syndrome represents a new way that biomedical researchers could construct scientific knowledge about racial difference. I show how metabolic syndrome became a racial project, an unfolding process that drew on different racial meanings to make sense of human metabolic difference and simultaneously used race to classify bodies and populations. Grounded in a critical race framework, I believe that metabolic syndrome seems to draw on earlier formations of race that link racial inequality to the essential properties of purportedly biologically and genetically meaningful groups. Second, metabolic syndrome was also forged in the context of biomedicalization, which encompassed an increasingly biological and technological approach to the study of human metabolism. Biomedical researchers and institutions combine new forms of molecularization, risk assessment, and population surveillance to produce ideas about racial difference and metabolic syndrome. Finally, the framework of biopower provides a way to think about how scientific disciplines such as demography and epidemiology, and emerging biomedical specialties such as cardiology and endocrinology, combined with government regulations on race and prescription drugs to create a racial context through which metabolic syndrome could emerge. The relations of biopower that encapsulate both metabolic syndrome and race discipline bodies and regulate populations so that they can be more easily targeted for biomedical research, political utility, and economic exploitation.

Chapters 2 and 3 narrate the emergence of metabolic syndrome and analyze how racial meanings were central to its construction. In chapter 2, "The Emergence of Metabolic Syndrome," I trace key moments in the social history of biomedicine when scientists and medical doctors began to create technologies for measuring the body's metabolic processes, examined these processes at the level of populations, and constructed theories that aimed to explain group differences in metabolic problems. I show how these processes, taken together, provided a context for metabolic syndrome to emerge in biomedicine and established a racial framework that scientists deploy to explain metabolic difference. Across these periods, I demonstrate that metabolic syndrome has had several different names and empirical definitions, each with different implications for how the syndrome constructs racial meanings and explains racial inequality.

In chapter 3, "The Scientific Racism of Metabolism," I show how race became a way of interpreting metabolic differences across individuals and social groups that is consistent with historical forms of scientific racism. I trace the production of racial meaning through three conceptual periods of the emergence of metabolic syndrome and show how in some historical moments this racial production is explicit and in others is implicitly woven into the everyday practices of biomedical science.

In chapters 4 and 5, I place African Americans at the center of my analysis and examine the discourses and practices that target their metabolism of prescription drugs and sugar. Once metabolic syndrome became an object that scientists could study, it traveled from the domain of scientific discovery to the domains of drug treatment and nutritional interventions. Just as the causes of metabolic syndrome are framed in racial terms that uphold biological constructions of African Americans' health problems, so are potential drug treatments and nutritional health interventions. In chapter 4, "Killer Applications: The Racial Pharmacology of Prescription Drugs," I investigate the use of race and metabolic syndrome in biomedical research on prescription drugs and African Americans and develop the metaphor of killer applications to examine how prescription drugs operate in the politics of metabolism. A killer application is a superior technology that combines human and nonhuman elements that structure bodily practices in a wide range of social, commercial, and scientific contexts: prescription drugs have become the new killer applications in biomedicine. I argue that the search for killer applications has transformed the ways that pharmaceutical corporations study prescription drugs, metabolism, and race. I interpret the ways that prescription drug research constructs and explains African Americans' relationship to metabolic syndrome through a comparative analysis of two specific drug classes that are differently related to the syndrome (statins and antipsychotics) and have become killer applications for particular health problems. I argue that race and metabolic syndrome intersect in unique ways in the racial pharmacology of these two potential killer applications. The case of statins involves the development and marketing of statins in populations with high cholesterol. The case of antipsychotics involves the pharmacokinetic effects that atypical antipsychotics have on the development of metabolic syndrome, explicitly in populations with schizophrenia. While equitable access to prescription drugs may constitute one partial remedy to racial inequalities in metabolic health, research findings in prescription drug research suggest that members of different racial groups might require different dosages or routes of administration of drugs, or perhaps different compounds altogether, based on the assumption that race is biological and genetic. This research, and the assumptions about race that uphold it, is consistent with a new approach in the pharmaceutical industry that creates and targets niche markets for killer applications that can treat multiple health problems simultaneously, or avoid the harmful side effects of existing medications.

Chapter 5, "Sugar Stained with Blood: African Americans, Sugar, and Modern Agriculture," links with the argument in chapter 4 to examine how sugar has served as the site of African American biopolitics. It is not possible to provide a critical interpretation of the politics of metabolism without recognizing and acknowledging the synergistic relationships between food politics and metabolic health problems. As elements of food regime organized through agricultural capitalism, the production and consumption of sugar have served to subordinate African Americans' bodies. I show how the construction of African Americans' metabolic processes as biological and genetic, and the promotion of individualist and culturalist understandings of African Americans' consumption of sugar, often take place absent a contextualized discussion about how technoscientific and capitalist shifts in the industrial production of sugar have impacted human metabolism. The significance of food politics is also apparent in stark contrast to the deployment of killer applications and the cultural power that prescription drugs have over people's metabolic lives. Indeed, the economic interests of food and drug companies operate in our bodies and shape the politics of metabolism in ways that go beyond posing food and drugs as disconnected political issues.

In the Conclusion, "Metabolic Insurrection," I review the book's main arguments and discuss the implications of these arguments for how we study and, possibly, resist the politics of metabolism. Contrary to the biopolitical logic of metabolic syndrome, human metabolism is not, and has never been, a strictly biological phenomenon that can be neatly attached to bodies and understood as disconnected from the social world. Rather, metabolism is a site for the kind of biopolitics that simultaneously manufactures health problems and their remedies, deploys race as a way of concealing inequality, and constructs powerful ideas like metabolic syndrome to sever the relationship between body and society. The Conclusion shows how the arguments presented contribute to and develop the existing critical research on scientific racism, color blindness, and biopolitics. If, as a society, we decided to invest in the sustainable production of foods that promote good metabolic health, as opposed to more and more killer applications, perhaps the politics of metabolism could begin to establish a context for human flourishing.

Metabolic Syndrome as a Fetishized Commodity

Drawing on Karl Marx's idea of a fetishized commodity within our experience in capitalist technoscience, it is hard to imagine at this point a more unabashedly constructed thing-in-itself designed for the purpose of profit. Acting with the authority of scientific, state, and corporate power, social actors called metabolic syndrome into existence in the government database, the corporate market report, and the physiological substrata of bodies and populations. As a consequence of living within a capitalist society, Marx writes:

> the productions of the human brain appear as independent beings
> endowed with life, and enter into relation both with one another and
> the human race. So it is in the world of commodities with the products
> of men's hands.[46]

Once people produce commodities, they begin to treat them as if they are alive and act in the world; to treat commodities this way is to fetishize them. Biologist and feminist science studies scholar Donna Haraway argues that "fetishism is about interesting 'mistakes'—really denials— where a fixed thing substitutes for the doings of power-differentiated lively beings on which and on whom, in my view, everything actually depends."[47] The fact that social actors have called metabolic syndrome into being does not mean that it exists in the world.

The metabolic fetish connotes the denial, disavowal, and error that undergird its social construction and racial meanings within the politics of metabolism. The names, definitions, and biomedical theories of metabolic syndrome have indeed changed over time, and for this reason the discursive formation of metabolic syndrome has never been consistent with itself. The term "metabolic syndrome" cannot contain the complexity of its history and those social actors who participated in manufacturing this complexity cannot contain its heterogeneously productive effects. Introducing the syndrome as a fetishized commodity helps to explain how this biomedical idea, this epidemiological finding, this marketing device, has become a new bright object within the biomedical gaze. The reified heat of the syndrome glows as brightly and as fleetingly as a shooting star, and biomedical scientists, corporate benefactors, and government agencies have been unable to avert their eyes from it. Metabolic syndrome is a discourse whose meanings and applications vary widely across biomedical, political, and commercial contexts.[48]

In the pages that follow, I develop a critical relationship to the knowledge-making practices that have produced a viable epistemological and racial framework for metabolic syndrome that has afforded it a provisional legitimacy in the world of scientific objects. Scientists have constructed an epistemological framework in which claims about metabolic syndrome have meaning for social actors and institutions that have an interest in the truth and validity of such claims. How can scientists, doctors, and patients know anything about metabolic syndrome? If a body meets the criteria for metabolic syndrome, does it "have" metabolic syndrome? How do social conditions within our politics of metabolism produce metabolic syndrome in bodies, and what can be done to bodies when they are said to "have" metabolic syndrome? Whether metabolic syndrome construct will be widely adopted by practicing physicians to diagnose patients is not clear. However, the inclusion of a diagnostic code for metabolic syndrome in the International Classification of Disease certainly signals that physicians and health-care institutions, like insurance companies, would be operating within accepted practices if they started classifying patients using this new category. Also not clear is what a diagnosis of metabolic syndrome would actually mean for patients, physicians, and the practice of medicine. What is clear is that metabolic syndrome has the potential to revolutionize the way that biomedicine conceptualizes, investigates, and intervenes on metabolic health problems by illuminating the interrelationships and processes that link metabolism to race.

CHAPTER ONE

Race, Biomedicine, and Health Injustice

Blood Sugar investigates the network of social, medical, and political relationships that have forged a link between metabolic syndrome and race in the United States. Recall the three questions that guide my argument. First, how did metabolic syndrome become a discourse and a technique for producing biomedical knowledge? Second, how are current conceptions and meanings of race and racial difference forged through the discourses and practices of metabolic syndrome? Third, what are the implications of this emerging relationship between metabolic syndrome and race for understanding the construction of racial meaning in the politics of metabolism? To situate these questions in broader intellectual contexts, I draw upon core ideas from three critical social theories—critical race theory, biomedicalization, and the social theory of Michel Foucault, especially his framework of biopower—to provide a synthetic framework that I use to interpret the politics of metabolism broadly and the relationships between metabolic syndrome and race in particular. These critical social theories provide several unique insights as to how metabolic syndrome and race operate together in the politics of metabolism.

Critical social theories encompass bodies of knowledge and sets of institutional practices that actively grapple with the central questions facing groups of people differently placed in specific political, social, and historical contexts characterized by injustice.[1] Critical social theories are committed to producing ideas and engaging in practices that serve the interests of social justice. The commitment to social justice expressed in *Blood Sugar* involves linking an analysis of institutionalized forms of racial inequality and racial health disparities to a discursive analysis of racial meaning in biomedical constructions of metabolic syndrome.

Scholars within these traditions have focused on how particular social institutions such as governments, corporations, and science shape the life chances of people and have worked to illuminate the social and political conditions necessary for fostering a more just society. This focus on justice stems from a shared understanding about the nature of modern forms of power that have structured social stratification and inequalities that predominate in Western societies. Moreover, each of these bodies of knowledge draws upon a political orientation to the production of scholarship that recognizes that objective intellectual production does not, and cannot, occur in an unequal and highly stratified society. Major works in each of these areas have analyzed the role of scientists and scientific practices in the formation of unjust social arrangements and have deconstructed those forms of knowledge that undergird those arrangements. In the following sections, I consider how each framework sheds light on different aspects of the relationships between race, biomedicine, and power, which together form an important theoretical context through which the politics of metabolism plays out in the United States. I conclude by outlining some of the areas of convergence, divergence, and synthesis across these theoretical frameworks.

The Framework of Critical Race Theory

Because critical race theory provides a framework for analyzing metabolic syndrome as a site for the production of racial meaning and enactment of racist practices within American society, it is important to outline some of its distinguishing ideas. While there are many different critical race theories that are linked to particular authors and research traditions within an array of academic disciplines and professional activities, in this section I speak about critical race theory as a more or less coherent body of scholarship that aims to interrogate and contest the discourses, ideologies, and social structures that produce and maintain conditions of racial injustice. Critical race theories analyze how race and racism are institutions that structure global, national, and local social formations and shape the life experiences of people living in racialized societies.

Critical race theories understand race as a constitutive feature of global social, political, economic, and cultural organization since the 1600s and not as a naturalized system of biological essences. Racial formation theorists Michael Omi and Howard Winant defined race as "a concept that signifies and symbolizes sociopolitical conflicts and interests in reference to different types of human bodies."[2] This definition reflects the centrality of the body to critical racial theories, because black and brown bodies have borne the brunt of racism. Race concepts and their accompanying racisms were used to establish colonial social systems, modern nation-states and global political economies, and the human biological sciences and medicine of the eighteenth, nineteenth, and twentieth centuries.[3]

Critical race theories understand racism as a vast and complicated system of institutionalized practices that structure the allocation of social, economic, and political power in unjust and racially coded ways. While some race theorists have examined racism as a form of maligned individual prejudice, critical race theorists tend to embrace a more institutional understanding of racism that aims to identify how racism is embedded in the racially patterned practices of social institutions.[4] In examining the institutionalized aspects of racism, critical race theories challenge the idea that people of color are responsible for their own oppression.[5] These theories continue to challenge entrenched racial inequalities in health, education, criminal (in)justice, political representation, and social class.[6] This body of knowledge is too broad to review in great detail here, so in the section that follows, I develop four themes from critical race theory that inform this book: (1) racial formation and racial projects; (2) science and medicine as sites of racial formation; (3) a focus on analyzing forms of scientific racism; and (4) the nation-state as a site of racial formation in the context of biomedical research.

Racial formation refers to the social and historical processes by which racial categories are created, transformed, and destroyed.[7] Racial formation theory emerged in the 1990s in response to contemporaneous theories of race that viewed race as an epiphenomenon of ethnicity, social class, or nationality. From this perspective, interpreting the meaning of race analytically in the context of racial formation involves framing race social-structurally and interpreting the racial dimensions in social structures.[8] For example, analyzing race in the context of criminal justice would involve examining how the laws and practices of social institutions structure the unequal treatment of racially categorized individuals, not just comparing statistical rates of incarceration across groups or conducting psychological experiments to determine the inherent criminality of prisoners. Race and racism, then, must always be understood in the context of the institutional relationships that are brought to bear in shaping racial conflicts and interests. In this way, the notion of racial projects is also central to racial formation theory because it articulates how discursive and institutional elements of race work together in the process of racial formation. According to Omi and Winant, a racial project is "simultaneously an interpretation, representation, or explanation of racial dynamics, and an effort to organize and distribute resources along particular racial lines."[9] Racial projects combine what race means in a particular discursive practice and the ways in which both social structures and everyday experiences are racially organized based on that meaning.[10]

A second major idea from critical race theory is the recognition of science and medicine as central to the construction of racial concepts and meanings that in turn influence the practices of social institutions across multiple levels of society.[11] As many critical race scholars have observed, the meaning of race in the context of science and medicine has shifted dramatically over the past century.[12] The very categories of normal science that appeared to be value-neutral were in fact laden with racial meaning. Scientific knowledge did not just reflect racism—Western science was an active participant in constructing and maintaining racism. In other words, Western science upheld racial projects but also itself depended on racial thinking. Normal science is seen as racist based on its history of collaboration with core social institutions such as the state, schools, the medical establishment, and insurance industries.[13] Critical race theorists challenged the scientific objectivity of race concepts arguing that because scientific knowledge production was complicit with institutional structures of racial power, it was incapable of producing an objective science of race, but could at best produce racial narratives or "fictions."[14] For example, critical race analyses have shown how eugenicists and statisticians worked to develop racist state policies and eugenics programs.[15]

In the wake of World War I, scientific meanings of race began to shift from the typological view to a population-based conception of race that has dominated biological theory.[16] In the typological view of race, every conceivable physical and mental characteristic of the human body was measured and compared across racial types in an effort to validate preexisting racial taxonomies. In the population view of race, anthropomorphic, mental, and social characteristics were compared across population groups classified into races to perform the same ideological work, to confirm the hardness and impermeability of racial categories. The population approach to race did not replace the typological approach, nor did the concept of population first emerge during this period following World War II; rather, race was increasingly conceptualized as a population phenomenon—a new way to talk about populations that are assumed to be different. Both typological and population-based explanations of racial difference can draw upon naturalist understandings of race. By the 1950s, the United Nations Educational, Scientific and Cultural Organization (UNESCO) statements on race signaled a new scientific consensus that race concepts were socially constructed and were without foundation in human biology or nature.[17]

Despite this new consensus view that human beings cannot be sorted into racial types or populations based on biological or genetic criteria, racial categories are still assumed to be proxies for genetic or biological variation in contemporary biomedical theory and practice.[18] Jennifer Reardon has astutely pointed out the pronouncement by UNESCO that race lacked scientific basis was not the watershed paradigm shift in racial science that many critical race theorists have assumed it to be.[19] Rather than having the effect of summarily excising race from scientific discourse and practice, this 1950 statement signaled the emergence of a science of race that was explicitly color-blind.[20] Whereas concepts of race had once formed the bedrock of human sciences, in the post-Holocaust context race was too politically charged to adequately serve the needs of geneticists, biologists, and anthropologists (and indeed sociologists) to appear not to be in service of scientific racism. The UNESCO statement further advises scientists and the public that to avoid the legacy of bad, ideologically corrupt racial science they should "drop the term race altogether and use the term *ethnic groups* [emphasis added]."[21] To remain consistent with broader efforts to promote a color-blind society, scientists in the post–World War II era followed UNESCO's prescriptions and devised their own strategies to avoid possible collusion with scientific racism. Commonsense notions of race as skin color were no longer thought of as objective, rational, or consistent with the newly affirmed role of science to liberate societies from destructive ideologies.

Relatedly, critical race theories have challenged racial projects that were used to create racial hierarchies and to justify white supremacy— these racial projects are called scientific racism. Scientific racism consists of scientific discourses and practices that served to explain and justify social inequalities as the natural outcome of hierarchically organized biological difference understood principally as racial difference. Scientific racism emerged as an ad hoc justification of colonial subjugation and slavery in the eighteenth century and is most readily associated with the social policies of eugenics and the Nazi racial holocaust in the nineteenth and early to mid-twentieth centuries. Racial formation theorist Howard Winant argues that scientific racism functions by severing the effects of racism from the causes of capitalist white supremacy by attributing systematic racial inequalities to the nature of things, namely, to science.[22]

Critical race theories have challenged scientific racism as a racial project by dismantling one of its core philosophical ideas: racial essentialism.
Racial projects can be defined as racist if they create or reproduce structures of racial oppression based on essentialist understandings of race.
Racial essentialism is the assumption that race categories reflect an inherent hierarchical organization of human bodies based on essences. It is the
philosophical underpinning of scientific racism because the presumptive
essential differences between populations are permanent and cannot be
caused by social forces. Racial essentialisms disallow institutional explanations of racism because they locate race within individual bodies, which
are always already classified into distinctive racial groups. In his analysis
of how European nation-states used race to justify colonial domination
and European expansion during the nineteenth and twentieth centuries,
philosopher of race David Theo Goldberg articulates a useful philosophical distinction between racial naturalism, racial primitivism, and racial
historicism that illustrates how different racial essentialisms operated in
the context of modern state formation.

Racial naturalism encompasses the idea that nature is the appropriate
medium through which to understand race and that racial inequalities,
therefore, are the product of nature. Through racial naturalism, race is
the conduit for collapsing what is social and historical into and upon
what is considered natural. For Goldberg, racial primitivism emerges
during the mid-twentieth century as a discursive bridge for racial essentialisms, as the forms of racial rule began to shift from racial naturalism toward historicism. As Goldberg explains, the logic of primitivism
was to transform the subjects of colonial subjugation into idealized ver-
sions of themselves, frozen in time and taken for granted.[23] In contrast to
naturalism and primitivism where non-Europeans are naturally inferior,
through racial historicism, racially subjugated peoples are historically
immature and are thus subject to the civilizing process that constituted
Manifest Destiny. Thus, racial historicism views racial inequality as the
outcome of history, a history guided by the hidden hand of Enlightenment
progress and modernity, the production of the "facts" of European racial
superiority.

Goldberg's analysis of the philosophical forms that racial essentialism
takes under conditions of modernity is importantly linked to his concept
of nation-states as racial states. The U.S. government is a central site of
racial formation, especially in terms of the knowledge-production apparatuses of the government that produce and enforce racial classification.[24] Since the taking of the first federal census in 1790, race has been

1. **American Indian or Alaska Native**: a person having origins in any of the original peoples of North and South America (including Central America) and who maintains tribal affiliation or community attachment.

2. **Asian**: a person having origins in any of the original peoples of the Far East, Southeast Asia, or the Indian subcontinent, including, for example, Cambodia, China, India, Japan, Korea, Malaysia, Pakistan, the Philippine Islands, Thailand, and Vietnam.

3. **Black or African American**: a person having origins in any of the black racial groups of Africa. Terms such as "Haitian" or "Negro" can be used in addition to "black" or "African American."

4. **Hispanic or Latino**: a person of Cuban, Mexican, Puerto Rican, South or Central American, or other Spanish culture or origin, regardless of race. The term "Spanish origin" can be used in addition to "Hispanic" or "Latino."

5. **Native Hawaiian or Pacific Islander**: a person having origins in any of the original peoples of Hawaii, Guam, Samoa, or other Pacific Islands.

6. **White**: a person having origins in any of the original peoples of Europe, the Middle East, or North Africa.

Figure 3. Racial and ethnic categories of the Office of Management and Budget, 1997.

a central feature of the United States' political data collection system. The 1790 census measured the numbers of "free white males" as well as the "the number of slaves."[25] For decades, the standard practice was for the census taker to make a determination as to the racial classification of individual members of the population. The federal government has employed numerous taxonomies of race in the census. In response to the changing terms and meanings of race and ethnicity used in federal data collection, in 1997 the Office of Management and Budget (OMB) issued new regulations on maintaining, collecting, and presenting federal data on race and ethnicity in the United States. The minimum categories for data on race and ethnicity for federal statistics, program administrative reporting, and civil-rights compliance reporting are defined in Figure 3. These regulations were intended to provide a standardized and universal language for defining the major population groups of the country and apply to all federal data collection efforts, including all clinical and bio-medical research funded by the government.[26] According to these regulations, the U.S. government and its agencies consider self-identification as the preferred means of obtaining information about an individual's race and/or ethnicity.

Nonetheless, the implementation of standardized federal racial and ethnic categories, and the technique of self-identification, permitted the continued expansion of recruitment of racial and ethnic groups into bio-medical research.[27] This represents a substantive shift from earlier forms of racial knowledge that were grounded in the institutions of science and medicine. Yet, the OMB states that its racial and ethnic categories were developed to represent social-political constructs and are not anthropologically or scientifically based. In other words, the federally mandated racial and ethnic categories are intended to be interpreted and applied in administrative and legal contexts, not scientific and biomedical contexts.

Sociologist Steve Epstein examined these and other recent changes in U.S. biomedical research policies and practices in the mid-1990s regarding the inclusion of racial and ethnic groups and women in clinical research and trials. Drawing on racial formation theory, he analyzes the U.S. government's regulation of racial categories in biomedical and clinical trials research. As of 1994, the National Institutes of Health policy was that women and members of minority groups and their subpopulation must be included in all NIH-supported biomedical and behavioral research projects involving human subjects.[28] Epstein's analysis raises important questions about what types of bodily difference the government should measure, how this measurement should be carried out, and how such differences should be interpreted.

Critical race theorists have focused on illuminating and contesting the social, economic, and political arrangements that undergird racism as a system of oppression. The themes I have outlined provide a sense of critical race theory's multiple interventions into these arrangements. Critical race theories have long recognized the centrality of science and medicine to the construction of racial concepts and meanings that in turn influence the practices of social institutions. Critical race theory provides an important theoretical framework because of this central preoccupation with the social reproduction of race and racism, particularly in American society. In the next section, I turn to the framework of biomedicalization to understand how recent shifts in science, medicine, and technology can help to account for the relationships between metabolic syndrome and race.

The Framework of Biomedicalization

The framework of biomedicalization constitutes a second important theoretical framework shaping this book. Biomedicalization is a historical and analytic framework for understanding the series of institutional, scientific, and technological processes that have transformed American bio-medicine on multiple levels of social organization, especially since the mid-1980s.[29] Whereas medicalization refers to a process whereby social practices, bodily processes, and bodily materials were subsumed under the jurisdiction of clinical medicine, biomedicalization refers to the ways that medicalization has been transformed by an increasingly biological and technological approach to medicine.[30] Biomedicalization has been theorized from within a broader interdisciplinary field called science and technology studies (STS). In elaborating the framework of biomedical-ization, I highlight five themes that are especially relevant to the argu-ments I make: (1) technoscience; (2) molecularization; (3) the increased importance of risk; (4) the development of biomedical capitalism; and (5) stratified biomedicalization.

The first idea from biomedicalization is technoscience, which is a way of understanding the practice of science as a social and cultural process.[31] This framing of the relationship between science and technology requires analyzing the practices by which scientific knowledges are culturally and collectively produced by scientists through their technologies—hence, technoscience.[32] Stated differently, scientists use technologies to manipu-late and interact with their objects of study in order to produce scientific knowledge. Scientific knowledge cannot be separated from the technolo-gies and social interactions that define the relationships between scientists and the material world. When applied to the field of biomedicine, this manipulation occurs through the use of biotechnologies such as diagnostic tools, screening tests, drugs, and other regulatory devices. Thus, an impor-tant understanding of technoscience, and one shared by many scholars in the field known as science and technology studies (STS), is that bio-medical scientists gain cultural authority and produce scientific objectivity by concealing the institutional practices that construct and constitute such knowledges and the unequal power relationships in which those techno-logical practices are embedded.

For example, in her Foucauldian-inspired analysis of the science of sex hormones, STS scholar Nelly Oudshoorn shows how cultural norms and ideas about sex difference shape the institutional practices that produce knowledge about masculine and feminine sex hormones. Whereas once the essential nature of femininity had been located in specific organs, espe-cially the uterus and the ovaries, Oudshoorn argues that with the techno-scientific interventions in the early twentieth century in organic chemistry, femininity increasingly became associated not with specific organs but with their chemical substances. She observes that prescientific ideas about sex difference influenced the interpretation of which hormones were la-beled as male and female. However, the social and cultural contexts in which these ideas about sex difference influenced knowledge produc-tion do not become part of the record of so-called scientific truth. The epistemology of technoscience recognizes the seamless relationships be-tween biomedical technologies, their bodily applications, and the scien-tific knowledge they are used to manufacture. "Science," Oudshoorn states plainly, "is not just words."[33]

As Oudshoorn's work on hormones suggests, a second theme of bio-medicalization is molecularization—the emergence and dominance of sci-entific practices, technologies, and theories that conceptualize and con-duct the surveillance of human life at the molecular level.[34] The cultural power of molecules such as DNA to define human difference became possible through molecularization and also through geneticization—the process through which differences between people are reduced to DNA codes.[35] Molecularization encompasses the processes of institutional and structural reorganization, the creation and application of new technolo-gies, and the production of new theoretical ideas about molecules and their relationship to human disease. Beginning in the late 1800s and con-tinuing to the present, molecularization was a central feature of the ways that the biological sciences conceptualized the body and its processes. The discovery of DNA and the flourishing of molecular biology in the 1950s provided technological and discursive resources for scientists to shift to-ward molecularization.

STS scholars have examined how scientists construct meanings of race at the molecular level. For instance, Sara Shostak analyzes two trends in genomic research on racial differences in environmental health that illus-trate this theme.[36] First, scientists in the fields of molecular epidemiology and toxicogenomics are measuring the effects of environmental expo-sures at the molecular level, that is, on DNA, genes, and gene expression. Second, scientists are using race to search for genetic differences that may shape individual and population responses to environmental exposures. On the one hand, these new molecular tools are viewed as enabling new strategies of disease prevention that might help to interrupt the process from environmental exposure to illness. On the other hand, these tech-niques might be used to create new scientific conceptions of race that sustain "a new era of molecularized scientific racism."[37]

A third theme from biomedicalization that emerges out of a techno-scientific approach to studying life at the molecular level is an increasing emphasis on risk in biomedicine. The so-called risk factor paradigm has been the dominant theoretical framework for chronic disease epidemiology since the second half of the twentieth century.[38] This methodological focus on risk in epidemiology reflects an influence of the dominant biomedical theory that human illness is caused by an interaction of environmental, physiological, and behavioral factors: so-called risk factors. In the risk factor paradigm, researchers produce risk statistics from population-level surveillance data that show that particular variables, often conceptualized at the molecular level, are statistically associated with an undesirable health outcome. Analysts then interpret these population-level risk statistics as individual-level risk factors that, by virtue of their expression of molecular processes, become transformed into biologically meaningful causes of poor health at the individual level. Practices of surveillance and discourses of risk are coproduced, which means that scientists use practices of surveillance to produce knowledge about risks, and then risks are used to justify further practices of surveillance.[39] In a racial context, as biomedical researchers analyze population surveillance data collected using race categories, these practices contribute to the construction of race as an individual-level cause of disease. In practice, race variables are often statistically associated with undesirable health outcomes, and in this context race is often interpreted as an individual-level risk factor. Marking bodies with risk *as* race suggests that race itself becomes an indicator of risk.

A fourth theme from biomedicalization that is relevant to this study is that biomedicine is a profitable global capitalist system that exploits human health as a commodity, especially the pharmaceutical industry.[40] Scholars such as Catherine Waldby and Nikolas Rose argue that contemporary biomedicine is increasingly driven and organized by the search for biovalue, or the production of a surplus out of life itself.[41] Feminist science studies scholar Charis Thompson takes this argument one step further to argue that biomedicine has helped to establish a new mode of capitalism in the United States—the biomedical mode of capitalist reproduction.[42]

Thompson identifies five distinguishing features of the biomedical model of reproduction that comprise biomedicalization as a capitalist system. First, whereas traditional forms of capitalism have focused on modes of production, biomedical capitalism has shifted to a focus on reproduction through the deployment of biotechnology. Second, as I suggested earlier, whereas traditional forms of capitalism produced profit through the extraction of surplus labor, biomedical capitalism has shifted to the extraction and maximization of profit out of bodies and their bodily products. Third, whereas traditional forms of capitalism alienated workers from their labor and the products of their labor, biomedical capitalism has shifted to a situation where bodies are alienated from the profits of their own reproduction. Fourth, whereas traditional capitalism is premised on the accumulation of capital in the present moment, biomedical capitalism is characterized by the success of procedures and processes that lead to promised future returns (e.g., developing future cures). Fifth, whereas traditional capitalism produced by-products or externalities that require disposal, the by-products of biomedical capitalism are often ethically sensitive materials (such as embryos) or are desirable in and of themselves (such as donated organs).

One central feature of the rise of biomedical capitalism is new biomedical–government–industry collaborations that involve the production, legitimation, and commercialization of biomedical knowledge.[43] These new relationships form the institutional bases out of which growing volumes of research are produced. For example, pharmaceutical companies pay academic biomedical researchers to conduct clinical trials for their new investigational drugs and then pay federal drug regulators at the Food and Drug Administration to review their drug for regulatory approval. In the context of a biomedical mode of capitalism and new ways of producing profitable biomedical knowledge, Sandra Soo-Jin Lee investigates the corporate research, development, and marketing of pharmaceutical drugs targeted at specific racial groups.[44] With regard to pharmaceuticals, Lee outlines what she calls an infrastructure for racialization, a set of scientific and institutional practices that inscribe bodies and their bodily products with racial meaning. These practices consist of (1) new research on human genetic variation that overlays genetic data onto social categories of race; (2) the continued and widespread use of race as a proxy for risk in clinical medicine; and (3) the commercial development of racially inscribed niche markets by the pharmaceutical industry.

The scholarship of Sara Shostak, Janet Shim, Charis Thompson, Sandra Soo-Jin Lee, and others suggests that the scientific, technological, and economic processes that encompass biomedicalization do not operate uniformly on all social groups. Thus, a fifth theme is that biomedicalization is a stratified and stratifying social process. Adele Clarke et al. define co-optative biomedicalization and exclusionary disciplining as two oppositional processes within biomedicalization that include and exclude particular bodies and populations from the domain of biomedicalization. Co-optative biomedicalization entails the expansion of medical jurisdiction over areas previously not deemed medical in terms of interventions targeted at particular social groups. For example, Sandra Soo-Jin Lee's work shows how racial groups are targeted in pharmaceutical development through the co-optation of race in biomedical research. Exclusionary disciplining refers to the institutionalized practices that erect barriers to the social process of biomedicalization for selected social groups. Drawing on my earlier example, members of racial and ethnic population groups who lack prescription drug coverage are excluded from the co-optative practices of pharmaceutical companies.

The framework of biomedicalization provides a set of powerful analytic tools with which to analyze the relationships of metabolic syndrome and race. In the next section, I turn to Foucault's framework of biopower. Biopower provides a synthetic conceptual framework for this book that views racial formation and biomedicalization as part of an overarching apparatus of power and knowledge.

The Framework of Biopower

The social theory of Michel Foucault, especially his analytic framework of biopower, provides a third and synthetic theoretical lens shaping this book. Foucault's framework of biopower contributes three important themes to this book. The first theme reflects a new emphasis on the relationships through which the life and health of populations become the objects of power and knowledge. The second theme recognizes that institutions of power use these techniques to organize and guarantee exploitative economic and political relationships. The third theme is that it specifies a Foucauldian theory of race and racism that emphasizes how biological and political relationships are deployed through racial categorization.

Foucault develops the concept of biopower as a way of understanding the transitional period beginning in the seventeenth century when modern institutions of power began to target human life as a political objective. The framework of biopower focuses on the relationships through which the life and health of bodies and populations become the objects of scientific discourse and institutional regulation by governments and corporations. Foucault conceived of biopower as the convergence of disciplinary power and a new kind of regulatory power over the life processes of entire populations, two "poles" of power that converge at the level of bodies and populations themselves.[45]

The first idea within a framework of biopower is that the two technologies of biopower, disciplinary power and regulatory power, represent distinct institutional locations for the operation of power and the production of knowledge. Disciplinary power is the means to extract political and economic productivity from individual bodies and the use of tactical procedures used to observe, judge, and examine bodies. Disciplinary knowledges are the scientific truths about the body produced through the observation, judgment, and examination of bodies. Achieving the discipline of the body requires hierarchical observation, normalizing judgment, and the physical examination.[46] Through these techniques and practices, disciplinary power establishes the relations of docility and utility of the body—this is how discipline makes docile bodies. Hierarchical observation involves the continuous and uniform monitoring of the processes of the body in order to achieve its maximal productive efficiency. Normalizing judgment involves the introduction of a system of rewards and punishments whose goal was to induce the body to conform to the laws of efficient movement corresponding to the activity it was being asked to perform under disciplinary conditions. The examination is the recurrent and culminating event in the disciplinary process through which the body is gazed upon as "both a ritual of power and a procedure for the establishment of truth."[47]

Whereas disciplinary power operates through strategies that target the individual body, regulatory power operates through "massifying" strategies that deal strictly with populations as "a political problem, as a biological problem, and as power's problem."[48] Regulatory power gained increasing prominence in the nineteenth century with the rise of demography, epidemiology, and sociology. The primary techniques of regulatory power involve the use of demographic averages, comprehensive and comparative measures, and statistical assessments that are derived from the surveillance of populations. Foucault provides the familiar example of the birthrate as such a measure. The birthrate is a statistical measurement that is used to evaluate the relative health of the population in terms of the number of live births in a given population over a given time period. In a recursive fashion, these measures are then used to establish further regulations that are intended to act on the population as a whole. If the birthrate is low, social interventions are required to improve the population's health. Whereas disciplinary power makes docile bodies so as to increase their utility, regulatory power acts through populations so as to maximize health and life.

Governments and corporations create and use these two forms of power to conform bodies and populations to unequal political and economic arrangements. With its explicit focus on the life processes of human populations, Foucault articulates biopower as a critique and synthesis of the

liberal-juridical and Marxist conceptions of power. The juridical or liberal conception of power maintains that the governments exercise the law
and the threat of death to rule over their subjects. Indeed, the nation-state
itself required the production of a discourse about a bounded population
of individuals—citizens. Foucault argues that governments had historically exercised their right to kill their enemies, both foreign and domestic,
and that this management of death was central to the extension of government power, especially military power. While governments continued
to kill and still do, during the transition to biopower governments began
to add a biopolitical approach to their repertoires. This new approach
was primarily concerned with investing in, interrogating, and controlling
the biologies of all living populations. To explain the significance of this
new political relationship, Foucault observes that "one might say that the
ancient right to *take* life or *let* live was replaced by a power to *foster* life
or *disallow* it to the point of death."[49]

A Marxist conception of power maintains that capitalists exercise
power to extract surplus value from the labor of workers. In contrast,
Foucault's conception of biopower maintains that scientific institutions,
governments, and corporations construct and deploy biological relationships for the economic regulation of populations. In Foucault's words,
biopower was central to the development and success of capitalism because it enabled "the adjustment of the phenomena of population to economic processes."[50] Modern capitalism requires the control of large numbers of individual bodies, not only in terms of a need for a population
of healthy laborers, but with the health of bodies as objects of political
investment and sources of economic revenue. The increasing commodification of health under biomedicalization is good evidence of this treatment of bodies and their products as sources of profit.

A third and crucial idea within the framework of biopower is that it
outlines a theory of race and racism. Foucault's published 1975–76 lectures at the Collège de France provide a unique elaboration of the concept
of biopower and its connections to the emergence of the concept of race
and the early formations of state racisms.[51] In these lectures, Foucault
argues that race emerged historically as a way to create a caesura—a
break—within the biological and population phenomena addressed by
biopower, a break used to separate out perceived biological risks to the
health and vitality of the population. For Foucault, race serves as a trans-
fer point between the production of biological knowledge about population health and the exercise of political power; race becomes a means of

"transcribing a political discourse into biological terms."[52] Thus, there existed a quick linkage between the exercise of biopower and nineteenth-century biological theories of race.[53]

Relations of biopower both enable and justify the practices of racism that have taken place in the name of strengthening or improving population health.[54] Modern racisms function in the context of biopower by establishing a perpetual relationship of war between races in which racial categorization emerges as a way to identify biological enemies, both internal and external, to a particular state government, and mark them for improvement, purification, or extermination. Given this framework, it is clear how and why racial discourses were deployed to institutionalize ideas and practices of population eugenics, which were presumably aimed at improving the health of populations through the purification of the racial stock.[55]

Issues of Convergence and Divergence

Thus far I have presented critical race theory, biomedicalization, and biopower as three distinctive bodies of scholarship that each offers unique contributions to *Blood Sugar* and to our understanding of race, biomedicine, and health injustice. However, sharp lines demarcating these areas are not so easily drawn as these areas have been shaped by and continue to influence each other in the broad context of critical social theory. While there are multiple points of convergence across these areas, they also diverge in meaningful ways that are germane to my synthetic interpretation of the relationships between metabolic syndrome and race.

A primary point of convergence across critical race theory, biomedicalization, and biopower is a focus on the multiple linkages between bodies and populations, and in particular how scientific ideas about the body emerge out of practices that are targeted at populations. Yet, within this convergence these three frameworks each treat this body–population link in different ways. Historically, in the United States, critical race theorists have been first and foremost concerned with the experiences of people of African descent living under unjust conditions of colonialism, slavery, and capitalism. The idea of race itself provided a pseudoscientific pretext for enacting various forms of racial subjugation under European rule that operated by linking ideas about the inferiority of particular racial types to population-based exploitations. In the same way, Foucault's thinking about race as a system of biopower draws upon this understanding of race but emphasizes how the operation of this new kind of power was enabled by a new focus on maximizing the life and health of dominant groups that emerged in the 1800s, nearly a century after the first racial taxonomies were codified in the European academy. Scholars in the field of STS more broadly begin their analysis of the body–population link with Foucault, accompanied by a heavy reliance on feminist ideas about the gendered body, and examine the multiple ways that bodies and populations are constituted via new technologies in science and medicine.

A second point of convergence concerns the research methods utilized to answer research questions in each area. Specifically, contemporary practitioners in critical race theory, biomedicalization, and biopower have all drawn upon discursive and historical methodologies to study different aspects of the relationships between power and knowledge. For example, in her book *Panic Diaries: A Genealogy of Panic Disorder,* sociologist Jackie Orr uses Foucault's genealogical method to analyze the relationships of power and knowledge developed by a normalizing society to regulate the psychological life, health, and disorders of individuals and entire populations—a concept she calls pychopower.[56] Drawing on Foucault's formulation of biopower, Orr argues that psychopower has emerged since the late nineteenth century but gained new operational capacities with the rise of twentieth-century information and communication technologies. She uses genealogy to identify three distinctive ways that the panic disorder serves as a site for the operation of psychopower. First, psychopower disciplines individuals and entire populations through the surveillance, scientific classification and management, and public administration of the psychic realms of perception, emotion, and memory. Second, the techniques of public-opinion polling, attitude measurement, and psychological testing both govern populations and have the effect of intensifying and multiplying the communicative feedback loops between governing bodies and the bodies they would govern. Third, by utilizing these new techniques and knowledges focused on perception, emotion, and memory, psychopower can blur the boundaries between the real and the unreal.

Through her articulation of psychopower, Orr contributes to a political understanding of how scientific practices and institutional relationships reproduce particular kinds of subjectivities and materialities. She shows how U.S. government propaganda about nuclear annihilation during the Cold War was informed by and proactively informed the social psychology of group trauma, fear, and panic, which were themselves financed by the state. She makes a similar genealogical argument about clinical trials for the antidepressant Xanax. The pharmacological effects of Xanax were tightly linked with the classificatory schema for panic disorder because of the new institutional relationships between biomedical psychiatry, the federal government (Department of Defense and FDA), and pharmaceutical corporations (Upjohn), which were the institutional locations for the classification, administration, and treatment of panic disorder.

While serving as an exemplar of a way to synthesize a framework of biopower in the context of science and technology studies, Orr's research also demonstrates a first point of divergence with critical race theory. While some critical race scholars draw upon Foucault's ideas (e.g., David Theo Goldberg) and the organizing principles of science and technology studies (e.g., Troy Duster), precious few Foucauldian and/or STS scholars draw upon the insights of critical race theory to address questions of race and racism in direct terms. Stated differently, these frameworks do not share equally across each other's domains of inquiry. A counterexample to this point of divergence is the work of Melbourne Tapper, who draws upon ideas about African American citizenship, medicalizing discourses about disease, and the operation of biopower to explore how sickle-cell anemia became an object of scientific intervention targeted on people of African descent.[57]

A second point of divergence across these areas concerns the use of different theoretical vocabularies to describe what I increasingly see as analogous social practices and arrangements regarding the reproduction of race and racism. For example, critical race theorists Michael Omi and Howard Winant advance the construct of racial formation to describe the processes by which racial categories are created, transformed, and destroyed. Racial formation, in their way of speaking, consists of the integration of the discursive meanings of race and the institutionalized practices of racism that function based on that meaning. In comparison, Michel Foucault advances a similar idea that race is reproduced through the convergence of the disciplining of bodies and the regulation of populations and that this reproduction takes place in order to propagate the unequal power and knowledge arrangements that comprise modern racisms. While it is likely that Omi and Winant were influenced by the so-called discursive turn in critical social theory popularized by Foucault, nonetheless, these two frameworks ostensibly describe the same social process using different linguistic formulations.

To conclude, these frameworks are synthetic because they help to identify the similar social process and institutional relationships that encompass the politics of metabolism. Figure 4 previews the themes I develop in this chapter and positions them relative to the core features of the politics of metabolism that I discussed in the Introduction: the social

	Critical race theory	Biomedicalization	Biopower
Social processes	unfolds via discursive and institutional processes	unfolds through synergies between technologies and science	reflects convergence of disciplines of the body and regulations of populations
Institutional relationships	biomedicine and nation-state as racial projects	new forms of biomedical–government–industry collaboration	frames relations between biomedical, state, and corporate institutions as political
Construction of racial meaning	race is constructed via process of racial formation	race is constructed in new structures of racial stratification	racial categorization constructs unequal scientific, political, and economic relationships
Construction of metabolic syndrome	new forms of scientific racism and racial essentialism	emphasis on molecularization and risk in the study and treatment of metabolic health	metabolic health of bodies and populations as new objects of power/knowledge

Figure 4. Theoretical themes and the politics of metabolism.

processes and institutional relationships that have linked race and metabolic syndrome. These frameworks highlight the relationships between biomedical scientists, the government, and corporations through which metabolic syndrome has emerged as a racialized phenomenon—namely, the social processes and institutional relationships of the politics of metabolism structure the emergence of metabolic syndrome and the construction of racial meaning. The social processes of racial formation and biomedicalization illustrate the combined use of racial categorization and biotechnologies to enact relations of biopower. The framework of biopower helps to reframe the institutional relationships between biomedical scientists, the government, and corporations that are involved in racial formation and biomedicalization. In the following chapters, I use the ideas summarized here to explore how metabolic syndrome emerged as a new discourse of biopower by tracing the technoscientific processes and institutional relationships that are involved in the production of new racial meanings. In the Conclusion, I address how my interpretation of the relationships between metabolic syndrome and race speak back to these theoretical frameworks.

CHAPTER TWO

The Emergence of Metabolic Syndrome

Years ago, I ordered the medical trade book *Contemporary Diagnosis and Management of the Metabolic Syndrome®* by Dr. Scott M. Grundy, a book that I suspected might be important for my interests in metabolic syndrome given its subject matter and author. Dr. Grundy is a leading figure in metabolic syndrome research and served as the chairperson for the National Cholesterol Education Program, the group responsible for institutionalizing metabolic syndrome in the federal health science structure. Medical trade books like this one are written principally for health providers to provide them with technical medical information that should aid in their daily work of treating patients. Published by Handbooks in Health Care Company, a division of the firm Associates in Medical Marketing Company Incorporated, this book is like nothing I had seen before. What I found in this book provided an important clue about the emergence of the metabolic syndrome: a drug information sheet for TriCor. When I first flipped through its pages, I found a sticker placed on its cover page that reads:

> This publication may contain information about unapproved uses of TriCor® (fenofibrate tablets) marketed by Abbott Laboratories. Please see accompanying TriCor full prescribing information. If you have any questions, please contact Medical Services at 1–800–633–9110.

TriCor is a prescription drug produced by Abbott Laboratories that patients can take to manage their cholesterol. Abbott Laboratories provided Associates in Medical Marketing Company Inc. with an education grant with the intent that this money would be used to produce "medical education" about metabolic syndrome.

Metabolic syndrome appeared in multiple sites of knowledge production in biomedicine and has taken different forms in these various sites over time.[1] The embodied and material phenomena that came to be called metabolic syndrome had different scientific names and empirical definitions, each representing disjunctures, moments when particular epistemological possibilities for scientific discovery are opened up and closed off. By using this construct of disjunctures, which represent the structure of discursive possibilities that emerge across sites of knowledge production, I show how this process of emergence does not result from conscious intentional choices on the part of biomedical scientists working in their respective fields. To the contrary, the social processes and institutional relationships that comprise the politics of metabolism seem to be more open-ended and heterogeneous and have created a set of possible conditions through which metabolic syndrome could emerge as a racial phenomenon in some historical moments, and seemingly nonracial in other moments.

This chapter is divided into three sections. The first section, "Creating Metabolic Subjects," highlights the early technical and conceptual work on bodies and populations, molecular processes, and clustering that shaped early meanings and practices of metabolic syndrome. The second section, "Establishing the Etiology of Metabolic Syndrome," follows the emergence of the syndrome through a second moment, where researchers advanced new ideas about the definition and causes of the syndrome. The third section, "The Ascendance of Metabolic Syndrome," chronicles a moment in the emergence of the syndrome, namely, when, in 2001, it comes under federal biomedical jurisdiction through the National Cholesterol Education Program and then accelerates out into the vast network of biomedical disciplines and research specialties. While these sections appear to be organized according to chronological time, each encapsulates discursive themes in the attempt to establish metabolic syndrome as a legitimate object of biomedical knowledge production and clinical intervention.

Creating Metabolic Subjects

During 1956–87, the technical and conceptual foundations of metabolic syndrome were tightly linked to three main sets of discourses and practices that operated in polyvalent fashion:[2] (1) the increasing technical focus on measuring the body's metabolic processes at the molecular level, (2) the institutionalization of metabolic surveillance of populations, and (3) the increasing conceptual focus on the clustering of metabolic risk factors that resulted from these practices. Taken together, these polyvalent discourses and practices comprise the technical and conceptual frameworks through which metabolic syndrome emerged as a new discourse and technique of biopower. By interpreting these technical and conceptual foundations of metabolic syndrome as elements of biopower, I explore how the syndrome emerged as a result of the synergy of molecularization and the risk factor paradigm in biomedicine—thus creating new metabolic subjects. In the sections that follow, I explain each of these technical and conceptual foundations in greater detail, highlighting how they each contributed to the emergence of metabolic syndrome.

The development of a range of techniques to measure metabolic processes within the body constitutes a first development during these moments that shaped the emergence of metabolic syndrome. Beginning in the mid-1800s and accelerating through the early 1900s, new scientific theories and concepts were developed and new technologies deployed to represent the body's metabolic processes at the molecular level. The creation of new technologies that would be used to study metabolism in terms of molecular processes, such as the discovery and synthesis of insulin in 1920, helped to reinforce the early scientific imperative to know more about how bodies metabolized compounds like glucose (more on this in chapter 5). The development of the technical apparatus used in physical examinations and laboratory tests made it technically and discursively possible to construct a metabolic syndrome. Figure 5 lists selected technical developments that contributed to metabolic syndrome between 1896 and 1998. Not only did these technologies structure the content of biomedical knowledge about metabolic processes of bodies at the molecular level, they also opened up and closed off particular possibilities in terms of the emergence of the syndrome. Once each of these technologies was in use, the embodied forms of data necessary for metabolic syndrome could be readily produced in laboratories, government health offices, and doctors' offices. Yet, the creation of technologies in a given historical moment delimits the technical aggregation of the various elements of the syndrome at later moments. In other words, the technical and conceptual foundations in this early period form a set of disjunctures that continue to structure the range of discursive possibilities for metabolic syndrome in the contemporary moment.

Metabolic process	Measurement	Technical development
blood pressure/ hypertension	systolic/ diastolic blood pressure measurement	1896 Riva-Rocci develops the mercury manometer. 1897 Hill and Bernard develop the aneroid manometer. 1904 Janeway publishes "The Clinical Study of Blood Pressure," which influences the medical director of Northwestern Mutual Life Insurance Company, Dr. J. W. Fisher, to include blood pressure in its physical examinations. By 1918, most insurance companies measured blood pressure in their examinations. 1917, 1921, 1927 American Bureau of Standards published major reports on the improvement and standardization of blood pressure measurement and equipment.
blood sugar/ insulin resistance glucose tolerance	fasting plasma glucose	1929 Horgaard and Thayssen develop what they call the insulin-tolerance test. 1983 DeFronzo, Ferrannini, and Koivisto develop the Eeuglycaemic hyperinsulinaemic clamp technique, the "gold standard" for measuring insulin resistance in vivo. 1985 Mathews and colleagues construct the homeostasis model assessment-insulin resistance index. 1998 Belfiore, Iannello, Volpicelli, and colleagues develop the oral glucose tolerance test.

Figure 5. Selected technical developments of metabolic syndrome, 1896–1998.

Metabolic process	Measurement	Technical development
cholesterol	LDL and VLDL triglycerides, HDL lipoprotein analysis	late 1800s origins of scientific studies of lipid metabolism 1948–present Framingham Heart Study was central to the establishment of the risk factor paradigm, especially regarding the role of total cholesterol in the development of cardiovascular disease (Kannel, McGee, and Gordon 1976). 1964 Konrad Bloch and Feodor Lynen are awarded the Nobel Prize in Physiology or Medicine for discoveries concerning the mechanism and regulation of the cholesterol and fatty acid metabolism. 1985 Goldstein and Brown receive a Nobel Prize for research on the cellular synthesis of cholesterol.
obesity	body mass index (weight in kg/ height in meters^2)	1942 Metropolitan Life Insurance Company issues weight-for-height tables that measure the "ideal weight" for men. 1959 MetLife includes women in its weight-for-height schema. 1980 USDA Dietary Guidelines for Americans attempt to standardize the measurement of body mass index, although the measurement of obesity would continue to undergo significant revision

Sources: Panteleimon A. Sarafidis and Peter M. Nilsson, "The Metabolic Syndrome: A Glance at Its History," Journal of Hypertension 24 (2006): 621–26; National High Blood Pressure Education Program and National Heart, Lung, and Blood Institute, "Summary Report: Working Meeting on Blood Pressure Measurement" (Bethesda, Md.: National Institutes of Health, 2002); Robert J. Kuczmarski and Katherine M. Flegal, "Criteria for Definition of Overweight in Transition: Background and Recommendations for the United States," American Journal of Clinical Nutrition 72 (2000): 1074–81.

A growing focus on measuring features of the body and the construction of certain ideas about particular populations based on these bodily measurements constituted a second important development during this period that enabled the subsequent development of metabolic syndrome. Take, for example, the work of University of Marseilles physician Jean Vague, who proposed an alternative anthropometric method that "traces the thickness of the fatty tissue on the surface of the body."[3] Vague becomes a central figure in this period and is routinely cited as one of the primary so-called fathers of metabolic syndrome concept because of his investigation of the causal relationships between obesity, heart disease, and diabetes.[4] His anthropometric method required the measurement, enumeration, and tabulation of the fatty tissue found at ten points on the trunk and limbs of the body. Vague articulates two hypotheses that illustrate the way he defined, measured, and interpreted these bodily measurements in relationship to sex difference. The first hypothesis is that "the relationship of the thickness of the fold of the nape of the neck to that of the sacral fold is much greater than unity in the normal male, but much less in the female."[5] The second hypothesis is that "the brachio-femoral adipo-muscular ratio, a comparison of the adipo-muscular ratio [the relationship between fat and muscle tissue] on the arm compared to the thigh, is above unity [greater than zero] in the normal adult female, while the inverse is true in the male" (21). He uses these measurements to construct a statistical representation of sex-differentiated obesities, an index of masculine differentiation (IMD). The IMD is "the average of the nape:sacrum ratio and the brachio-femoral adipo-muscular ratio" (ibid.). This information is significant because Vague developed a body of conceptual and technical language that emphasized the measurement of the body, and the statistical comparison of different parts of the body, that were essential to his ideas about bodily difference.

Vague's hypothesis proposes that the essential biological difference between men and women can be articulated through measurement and comparison at these locations of the body. Based on his analysis of six hundred subjects, he constructs five mutually exclusive groups, standardized around a value of "0" for the standard male body, comprising the following categories: "hyperandroid" (+15 IMD), "android" (+15 to –15 IMD), "intermediate" (–15 to –45 IMD), "gynoid" (–45 to –75 IMD), and "hypergynoid" (less than –75 IMD). These categories are meant as descriptions of the different types of distributions of obesity typically found in women and men, with android referring to men and gynoid to women. The binary logic of sex drives Vague's interpretations of his statistics. In this regard, he notes that "fat distribution is very definitely a sexual characteristic, but there is a high percentage of overlapping between one sex and the other, especially at the two extremes of life" (24). In other words, while the category gynoid is meant to refer to a particular construction of populations as sexed, men can present with gynoid forms of obesity and women with android forms of obesity.

Vague concedes the nonexclusive nature of his sexed categories as demonstrated by the images of his subjects, which were published in the *Journal of Clinical Nutrition*. The text of his paper was published along with several tables and figures, as well as eight photographs of four of his research subjects, whose bodies are fully exposed to show the visual distributions of their obesities. One image shows a woman and a man both classified with gynoid obesity, whereas the other shows a woman and a man both classified with android obesity. The images of Vague's subjects and the captions that accompany them represent the visual forms of bodily evidence that he used to present ideas. The captions note specific information about the subject's metabolism, including age, height, weight, blood pressure, the presence or absence of diabetes, and other bodily indicators, including hair, the status of genitals and sexual practices, and the subjects' value for the index of masculine differentiation. Undoubtedly, disciplinary conventions about publishing photographs of nude research subjects in professional biomedical journals have changed somewhat since the 1950s, but the visual representation of these subjects suggests the ease with which physicians might have differentiated between gynoid and android forms of obesity.

Vague's work illustrates the growing emphasis on measuring the body, but it also points to how specific ways of interpreting the bodily measurements begin to make metabolic syndrome possible. One important way Vague's ideas preview the emergence of metabolic syndrome lies in his claims about android obesity as a common cause of heart disease and diabetes. In this brief passage, he describes how android obesity is the common cause of atherosclerosis and diabetes:

> The inconstancy of diabetes in the course of atherosclerosis when the islets of Langerhans offer a sufficient genetic resistance to the overwork imposed by the pituitary-adrenal overactivity, in contrast to the constancy of atherosclerosis in adult diabetes and its relative independence to the degree of hyperglycemia, cease to surprise us if we regard arterial legions and diabetes as the consequences of an identical cause

[android obesity] acting against a backdrop which may suffer from a genetic fragility of the islets or be free from it.[6]

In other words, Vague posited that heart disease and diabetes share android obesity as a common cause. According to him, the development of diabetes, gout, uric calculous disease, and atherosclerosis is "very strongly favored by android obesity, especially when weight and the index of masculine differentiation are very high" (29). In contrast, gynoid obesity "does not exercise any direct influence on the metabolic disorders" (ibid.). In Vague's thinking, genetic differences between bodies caused both the differential development of android obesity and, consequently, diabetes and heart disease.

A second important way Vague's ideas preview the syndrome lies in the predictive power he attaches to the statistical construct, the IMD, for classifying bodies that are likely to develop metabolic disease. By 1956, he proposed that a particular combination of bodily measurements results in the best statistical predictor of android obesity. Stated differently, Vague's method was significant because it represented an important shift from diagnosing the body through physical examination to aggregating the results of individual-level physical examinations to construct statistical ideas about population-based risks. In other words, the IMD is a statistical construction that successfully identifies obese bodies that are predisposed to diabetes and to heart disease because of a theoretical common genetic mechanism. He states that the index of masculine differentiation has "always indicated to us the exact position of these forms [of obesity] in our classification and, in addition, has provided prognostic data" (24). His hope was that physicians would calculate the IMD and use it to predict—with great accuracy, in his view—which bodies and populations are likely to develop metabolic disease.

Increasing reliance on the notion of clustering to guide biomedical research on metabolism constitutes a third important development during this period that enabled the emergence of metabolic syndrome. Clustering refers to the observation that several different metabolic conditions are more likely to occur together in one individual than would be expected by chance alone. The notion of clustering is significant because the production of knowledge about metabolic syndrome is made possible by the physical examination and biochemical surveillance of bodies and the aggregation of those individual-level biological data to the level of populations. These conceptual developments in epidemiology are directly linked to the technical and conceptual foundations of metabolic syndrome because of the widespread use of metabolic syndrome as a statistical predictor of heart disease and stroke in biomedical research.

In the early 1920s, several German physicians were the first to document and publish research about the clustering of metabolic problems they observed in their patients, and the potential risks such clustering could pose to metabolic health.[7] Although none of these physicians explicitly codified a syndrome, they had similar theoretical ideas about how different metabolic processes worked together in the body. For example, in his 1936 study of insulin action, endocrinologist H. P. Himsworth created the distinction between insulin sensitivity and insensitivity, the latter being most likely to precede and then accompany the development of type 2 diabetes.[8]

While the focus on measuring the body's metabolic processes in terms of clustering represented a shift in the biomedical approach to studying metabolic states, it also formed the basis of later struggles to subsume metabolic syndrome under different disciplinary specialties. For example, Himsworth's research on insulin metabolism in the 1930s anchored the structure of contemporary endocrinology, and the efforts of contemporary endocrinologists to study metabolic syndrome make sense given this technical and conceptual anchor. Early scholars, like Vague, drew explicitly upon notions of risk-based clustering in their theories about the nature of metabolic problems, but it was not always with respect to the same outcome. Whatever the outcome, these notions of clustering formed the logic on which risk-based syndromes, such as metabolic syndrome, would be constructed in later decades. Different clusters of conditions drew the attention of newly developing medical specialties such as endocrinology and cardiology. In this early period, endocrinologists were concerned mostly with glucose metabolism, insulin, and diabetes; cardiologists were concerned with heart disease and the processes underpinning vascular function; rheumatologists were concerned with gout; and so on. Increasingly, over this thematic period, physicians would continue to conduct clinical research on the interrelationships between basic metabolic processes with a growing list of new molecular compounds and physical examinations.

While many of these early metabolic researchers developed and used statistical methods of analysis in their clinical research, in the late 1940s, the U.S. federal government assumed a new role in producing information about the metabolic health of populations. Indeed, the incorporation of a population approach to metabolism represents a major disjuncture in the emergence of metabolic syndrome. In epidemiology, the statistical computation of disease incidence and prevalence is made possible only through the numerical comparison of individuals within a defined population. In 1948, the National Heart Institute provided funding for the Framingham Heart Study, the first population heart study to include all of the physical exams and laboratory tests required to make a classification of metabolic syndrome in the United States.[9] The Framingham study is also noteworthy for its role in identifying cholesterol as a so-called risk factor in the development of heart disease. Following the successes of the Framingham study at identifying risk factors for heart disease, the U.S. Congress passed the National Health Survey Act of 1956, which authorized "a continuing survey and special studies to secure accurate and current statistical information on the amount, distribution, and effects of illness and disability in the U.S. and the services rendered for such conditions."[10] According to the National Health Survey Act of 1956, the empirical data for these new government studies would be drawn from at least three sources: (1) the people themselves by direct interview, (2) clinical tests, measurements, and physical examinations on sample persons, and (3) places where persons received medical care such as hospitals, clinics, and doctors' offices.

This law was significant because it mandated that the government conduct routine surveillance of its populations by use of physical examinations and laboratory tests that had hitherto focused on individual bodies. This act led to the creation of the National Health Interview Survey (NHIS), first conducted in 1957, the National Health Examination Survey (NHES) beginning in 1960, and the National Health and Nutrition Examination Survey (NHANES), which began in 1967. The NHANES study is the population study the National Cholesterol Education Program (NCEP) analyzed in its postulation of metabolic syndrome in 2001. These government studies have been and remain the largest population health surveys conducted in the United States each year. Thus, population health studies over the next five decades were designed using the Framingham study as a gold-standard model.[11]

These two conceptual and technical developments, one set focused on individual bodies and the other on populations, converge in risk-based syndromes. Risk-based syndromes are sites where ideas and practices about molecular processes, bodies and populations, and clustering come together in a polyvalent fashion. For example, the International Diabetes Federation (IDF) published its own version of metabolic syndrome and drew upon a definition of syndrome from a 1995 dictionary of epidemiology, which states that what distinguishes syndromes from diseases is their lack of a clearly defined cause.[12] It notes:

> A syndrome is defined as a recognizable complex of symptoms and physical or biochemical findings for which a direct cause is not understood. With a syndrome, the components coexist more frequently than would be expected by chance alone. When causal mechanisms are identified, the syndrome becomes a disease.[13]

Currently, the National Library of Medicine's online medical dictionary defines a syndrome as "a group of signs and symptoms that occur together and characterize a particular abnormality."[14]

Throughout the 1960s and into the 1970s, given the increasing proliferation of biomedical laboratories across the United States and the increasing availability of epidemiological data, more researchers would have access to the technologies and interpretative frameworks necessary to produce knowledge about risk-based syndromes. The 1960s saw several noteworthy contributions to the emergence of metabolic syndrome, but still unresolved was the semantic issue of what to call the syndrome, and which factors to include in its definition. In 1966, French researcher J. P. Camus theorized that gout, diabetes, and hyperlipidemia comprised "a metabolic trisyndrome."[15] The following year, Italian researchers advanced the notion of a "plurimetabolic syndrome" that included diabetes, obesity, and hyperlipidemia.[16] And in 1968, German researchers published an article in a prominent German medical journal about the interrelationships between hypertension and diabetes.[17]

It was during the 1970s that the specific term "metabolic syndrome" first appeared in the biomedical research literature. In 1976, Gerald Phillips, drawing heavily on Vague's work, theorized that the "constellation of abnormalities" that comprised increased heart disease risk could be explained by sex hormones.[18] In 1977, three studies were published that each codified specific formations of "metabolic syndrome" into the biomedical literature.[19] A few years later, in 1981, two German researchers were also among the first to publish research on "metabolic syndrome."[20] While the names and empirical definition of metabolic syndrome would continue to change in the coming years, the increasing scientific focus on the clustering of conditions in bodies and populations was made possible by new biomedical technologies.

The different names, definitions, and disciplinary origins for metabolic syndrome represent disjunctures in the emergence of the syndrome. The incommensurability of the syndrome across cardiology, endocrinology, and epidemiology meant that there would continue to be struggles over its name and meanings in biomedicine. Indeed, much of the controversy that appears in biomedical journals has been over the name, empirical definition, and predictive power of the syndrome concept. These debates about names, definitions, and statistics are important, but not what is most central about the technical and conceptual apparatus of metabolic syndrome. The technologies and conceptual developments that undergird the syndrome made it possible for it to travel across these disciplinary boundaries with remarkable ease. For example, nearly all medical practitioners and biomedical researchers, regardless of specialty area, have access to and widely utilize technologies that produce measurements of blood pressure, blood sugar, and obesity. They are ubiquitous in American biomedicine. These metabolic technologies were readily adaptable in different biomedical contexts from government public health offices and doctors' offices to people's own homes.

Yet, when these same researchers study metabolic syndrome within the confines of their own respective areas, it becomes possible for them to insert and/or omit particular features of human metabolism that are deemed relevant or irrelevant to their biomedical perspective. Issues about the technologies to use in crafting the syndrome's empirical definition are related to the effort to establish the syndrome as a disease with a cause. In order to make a transition from a syndrome into a disease, metabolic syndrome needed an identifiable biochemical and physiological mechanism, one that is interpretable only through the use of specific metabolic biotechnologies. In the next section, I explore how the search for a cause of metabolic syndrome inside of endocrinology reflects this kind of struggle.

Establishing the Etiology of Metabolic Syndrome

In a binomial equation, the letter "X" stands for an unknown variable that bears a measurable relationship to another known variable, "Y." In order to solve for Y in such an equation, the value of X must be known. This simple logic framed the second period of emergence of metabolic syndrome with physicians' efforts to take existing observations about the clustering of multiple risk factors (Y) and use them to construct new forms of knowledge about the causal interrelationships between these risk factors (X). Specifically, this period consisted of professional physicians, mostly endocrinologists, trying to advance new theories of what *caused* metabolic syndrome. Such theories were intended to help galvanize the syndrome as a biological disease and formal clinical diagnosis.

Perhaps by discovering the cause of metabolic syndrome ("X"), their logic suggested, researchers might then be able to discern the real value and meaning of metabolic syndrome ("Z"). During this period, different research groups hoped to explain the statistical associations between heart disease risk factors with causal theories focused on metabolic syndrome. In other words, researchers made continued efforts to establish the cause—or etiology—of metabolic syndrome.

One major moment in this process occurred in 1988 when Dr. Gerald Reaven accepted the Banting Award, named in honor of Sir Fredrick Banting, who synthesized human insulin in 1920, and gave the Banting Lecture to the American Diabetes Association based on his research on the role of insulin resistance in the development of heart disease.[21] In this lecture, Reaven defined "syndrome X" as a series of six related variables that tend to occur in the same individual—resistance to insulin-stimulated glucose uptake, hyperglycemia, hyperinsulinemia, an increased plasma concentration of VLDL triglyceride, a decreased plasma concentration of HDL-cholesterol, and high blood pressure. Reaven's hypothesis is that insulin resistance is the common cause of the five other components of syndrome X, and therefore is a primary cause of heart disease. This framing of insulin resistance as the cause of syndrome X stands in stark contrast to Vague's earlier theory that android obesity was the cause of heart disease and diabetes, although Reaven did, in effect, identify a potential common cause of both diabetes and heart disease—insulin resistance. While the construct of syndrome X would not acquire the cache of metabolic syndrome, owing in part to his omission of obesity in its definition, Reaven's influence on the science of metabolic syndrome is noteworthy. Despite the existence of multiple methods for measuring insulin resistance, none has been institutionalized in population survey research to the extent that other biological measurements of diabetes have, such as fasting blood glucose, in large part because of their expense.[22]

Dr. Reaven's 1988 lecture surprisingly does not include a technical definition of syndrome X. Whereas Vague went to great lengths to include highly specific physiological measurements and statistical procedures in his codification of metabolic syndrome, Reaven's omission of these details represents a disjuncture in the emergence of the syndrome. Specifically, whereas clustering was the central conceptual anchor in the earlier thematic moment, in this moment the cultural power of biological causality serves to anchor and promote the truth properties of metabolic syndrome. In his published lecture, Reaven did not intend to establish a new statistical concept in the biomedical landscape. Instead, his introduction and reference to syndrome X are more of a passing reference to the unknown nature of these metabolic processes:

> Based on available data, it is possible to suggest that there is a series of related variables—syndrome X—that tends to occur in the same individual and may be of enormous importance in the genesis of coronary artery disease. These changes include resistance to insulin-stimulated glucose uptake (insulin resistance), hyperglycemia (glucose tolerance), hyperinsulinemia, increased very low-density lipoprotein (VLDL) triglyceride, a decreased plasma concentration of HDL-cholesterol, and high blood pressure.[23]

Whereas in 1988 Reaven's hypotheses about syndrome X were more tentative, by 2000 he was calling it "the silent killer." In his 2000 coauthored book *Syndrome X: The Silent Killer: The New Heart Disease Risk*, he metaphorically calls syndrome X "the silent killer," a not-so-subtle reference to the paradox that although the syndrome has no visible symptoms (he did not include obesity in his conceptualization), it may be responsible, he argues, for up to 50 percent of heart disease in the United States.[24] Because the book seems to have been written for a general audience, it includes a "Self-Assessment for Risk of Syndrome X" rather than a formal scientific definition.[25]

After Reaven's original hypothesis, what remained unknown, or at least unsettled, about the etiology of metabolic syndrome was more than made up for with the growing list of heart disease risk factors that were correlated with the syndrome. By the end of the 1990s, other groups of researchers advanced several similar constructions that aimed both to encapsulate these hidden physiological relationships and to challenge Reaven's syndrome X. These constructions all draw upon the early conceptual and technical foundations and propose different names and empirical definitions of risk-based syndromes: the deadly quartet, the insulin resistance syndrome, the multiple metabolic cardiovascular syndrome, the chronic cardiovascular risk factor clustering syndrome, and multiple metabolic syndrome.[26]

Perhaps the hope for each of these constructions was that they could become central to the subsequent development of a science of metabolic syndrome that would extend outside the domain of biomedical journals and conferences. The effort to institutionalize metabolic syndrome outside particular biomedical specialties got under way in the early 2000s. In 2000, the American Association of Clinical Endocrinologists secured a petition to have a diagnosis code assigned to "dysmetabolic syndrome X" in the World Health Organization's International Classification of Disease (ICD-9-CM).[27] This meant that physicians could now use a specific code, 277.7, to diagnosis dysmetabolic syndrome X in their patients. According to the new diagnostic criteria, dysmetabolic syndrome X is "a multifaceted syndrome characterized by hyperinsulinemia; dyslipidemia; essential hypertension; abdominal obesity; and glucose intolerance in individuals with insulin resistance."[28] With the codification of the dysmetabolic syndrome X in the ICD, what had started out for Reaven as an unknown with syndrome X could now be known through an institutional classification with a simple diagnostic code.

The Ascendance of Metabolic Syndrome

The third moment, which began in 2001 and continues into the present, is characterized by continued institutionalization within biomedicine over what metabolic syndrome is, what it means, and who gets to define it as a legitimate disease. The culmination of past disjunctures directly impacts the structure of contemporary institutional power struggles over the authority to produce a science of metabolic syndrome. In the broadest terms, whereas Vague had been fundamentally concerned with obesity and its multiple effects on metabolic health, and Reaven's work puts insulin resistance at the center of the analysis of syndrome X, the effort to establish metabolic syndrome as a derivative of cholesterol metabolism represents a defining disjuncture for metabolic syndrome. In this section, I explore the effort to institutionalize metabolic syndrome and analyze how earlier disjunctures shaped the subsequent ascendance of metabolic syndrome as a formal and legitimate object of biomedical knowledge and practice.

In 2001, what began as a multiyear, multiagency government effort to study cholesterol turned into a pivotal shift in the emergence of metabolic syndrome. The National Cholesterol Education Program (NCEP) began in 1985 as part of a National Heart, Lung, and Blood Institute (NHLBI) effort to examine the dynamics of high cholesterol among American adults. The NCEP brought together experts from across the government, universities, and professional medicine. Stated differently, the NCEP was an example of a biomedical–government–industry collaboration that, given its centrality in defining metabolic syndrome during this period, wielded significant influence in biomedical research on cholesterol and its relationship to heart disease.

In addition to publishing aggressive new standards for the clinical management of cholesterol, the NCEP defined metabolic syndrome by

calling it a *secondary* target of intervention in its final report.[29] By framing metabolic syndrome as a secondary target of intervention, the NCEP
argued that clinicians could not adequately address the heart disease risk
from high cholesterol without acknowledging the role additional risk factors played in the development of heart disease. Under this logic, codify-
ing the construct of metabolic syndrome was intended to make practicing
physicians aware of the need to address the clustering of risk factors for
heart disease in their patients.

According to the NCEP, in order to be classified with metabolic syndrome, a research subject would have to submit a blood sample (for analysis of cholesterols, fasting blood sugar, and other molecules) and submit
to a physical examination including measurement of blood pressure,
height, weight, and abdominal circumference. If the subject's levels met or
exceeded three of five predetermined empirical norms, the individual was
said to "have" metabolic syndrome. The five components and their values for the NCEP definition are (1) blood pressure (higher than 130/85);
(2) fasting blood sugar (higher than 110 mg/dl); (3) LDL or "bad" cholesterol (higher than 150 mg/dl); (4) HDL or "good" cholesterol (lower than
40 mg/dl for men and 50 mg/dl for women); (5) abdominal circumference
(greater than 40 inches for men and 35 for women).

However, framing the syndrome as a *secondary* target of intervention
seems to have had the unintended effect of signaling to the biomedical
research community, pharmaceutical corporations, and the government
itself that metabolic syndrome required special attention as a *primary* object of knowledge. In a 2003 meeting at the National Institutes of Health
on metabolic syndrome, Dr. Scott Grundy, the chairman of the NCEP,
reflected that because the group of scientists was "concerned that the
NCEP guidelines would be seen as only drug treatment guidelines for LDL
[cholesterol], they decided to define a set of medical conditions related
to obesity, physical inactivity, and nutrition and define these conditions
as a metabolic syndrome."[30] In other words, the NCEP's action to define
metabolic syndrome seems to have been a way to cloak the practice of
setting cholesterol control standards to drug regimes in a scientific garb.
I will return to the relationship of metabolic syndrome to pharmaceutical
capitalism in chapter 4.

The additional significance of this disjuncture is that, through the
NCEP's codification of metabolic syndrome, the syndrome came under
the province of government's scientific authority, opening up possibilities
for new streams of federal funding and research collaboration. Whereas
in earlier periods the syndrome had been debated among practicing

	Reaven's Syndrome X (1988)	World Health Organization: metabolic syndrome (1999)	National Cholesterol Education Program Adult Treatment Panel III: metabolic syndrome (2001)	American Association of Clinical Endocrinologists and American College of Endocrinology: Insulin Resistance Syndrome (2002)	American Heart Association and the National Heart, Lung, and Blood Institute: metabolic syndrome (2005)
Criteria	*all of the following*	*elevated glucose and dyslipidemia plus two or more of the following biomarkers*	*3 of 5 of any of the following biomarkers*	*all of the following*	*3 or more of 5 of the following*
Elevated blood sugar	insulin resistance	elevated glucose ≥ 110 mg/dl	elevated glucose > 110 mg/dl	excluding type 2 diabetes fasting glucose of 110–125 mg/dl or 2 hr postglucose (75g) > 140 mg/dl	elevated glucose ≥ 100 mg/dl or drug treatment for glucose
"Bad" LDL cholesterol dyslipidemia	increased VLDL	LDL triglycerides ≥ 150 mg/dl or HDL < 35 mg/dl	LDL triglycerides > 150 mg/dl	LDL triglycerides > 150 mg/dl	LDL triglycerides ≥ 150 mg/dl or drug treatment for cholesterol
"Good" HDL cholesterol	decreased HDL	LDL triglycerides ≥ 150 mg/dl or HDL < 35 mg/dl	HDL cholesterol men < 40 mg/dl women < 50 mg/dl	HDL cholesterol men < 40 mg/dl women < 50 mg/dl	HDL cholesterol men < 40 mg/dl women < 50 mg/dl
Blood pressure	high blood pressure	blood pressure > 160/90 or drug treatment for hypertension	blood pressure > 130/85	blood pressure > 130/85	blood pressure ≥ 130 systolic or 85 diastolic or drug treatment for hypertension
Obesity	not included	abdominal circumference weight/height ratio > .90 or BMI > 30 kg/m^2 or waist circumference ≥ 94 cm	abdominal circumference men > 40 inches women > 35 inches	body mass index (BMI) adjusted by ethnicity, waist circumference, and family history of type 2 diabetes	abdominal circumference men ≥ 102 cm women ≥ 88 cm
		also includes microalbuminuria or the urinary albumin excretion rate			

Figure 6. Selected major definitions of metabolic syndrome, 1988–2005.

physicians who specialized in endocrinology and cardiology, it would now—however conceptualized—be a major target of government health research and intervention. This moment is also significant because, despite the earlier ICD-9-CM classification for dysmetabolic syndrome X in 2000, as a result of the NCEP action, metabolic syndrome increasingly came to acquire significant currency across biomedicine.

The NCEP's definition of metabolic syndrome created both controversies and opportunities for research in the biomedical community. Partly in response to the NCEP definition, two years later the American Association for Clinical Endocrinologists and the American College of Endocrinology, which included Dr. Reaven, began a renewed campaign to use the construct "insulin resistance syndrome" instead of the NCEP's metabolic syndrome.[31] Dr. Reaven has continued to be a critical voice in the debates about metabolic syndrome and similar concepts, despite being a key member of the NCEP, and has advocated for the use of different terms at different times.[32] The critical issues in these controversies were over what specific biomarkers would be part of metabolic syndrome definitions and how scientists theorized the biochemical and physiological etiology of the syndrome. For example, including or excluding a particular biomarker has direct implications for the technologies that need to be available in clinical and epidemiological settings to conduct metabolic syndrome research. Also, the inclusion and/or exclusion of biomarkers reclassifies which individuals and groups are defined as having the syndrome.

To add to the ongoing struggles to name and define the syndrome, funded by an educational grant from AstraZeneca pharmaceuticals, the International Diabetes Foundation (IDF) convened a 2004 workshop consisting of twenty-one experts in the fields of diabetes, public health, epidemiology, lipidology, genetics, metabolism, nutrition, and cardiology.[33] The workshop aimed to establish a new unified definition of metabolic syndrome that could be used to compare different populations around the world.[34] It presents several different hypothetical causes of metabolic syndrome: insulin resistance, obesity, genetic profile, physical inactivity, aging, and a proinflammatory state.[35]

In 2005, the NCEP and the American Heart Association (AHA) published an official statement affirming metabolic syndrome as a useful and valid construct.[36] The NCEP/AHA grounded this affirmation in their view that metabolic syndrome clinically identifies a person at increased risk for cardiovascular disease and/or type 2 diabetes mellitus.[37] However, what is significant about their defense of the syndrome is that they argue that the *clinical* significance of metabolic syndrome comes through its power as an indicator of statistical risk of disease, not through its existence as a disease with a unique pathogenesis. Yet, the authors argue that getting "a better understanding of the cause(s) of the syndrome may provide an improved estimate for developing ASCVD or type 2 diabetes for individuals."[38]

These discourses about metabolic syndrome signal that the long-standing cultural power attached to diseases with known biological causes has accompanied, and perhaps in some way was supplanted by, the increasing influence of risk-based syndromes with predictive power. It seems that metabolic syndrome might become the first disease without a known cause. The disjuncture in this discursive moment is that after risk-based syndromes are identified via statistical manipulation, scientists then work to uncover the assumed-to-exist biological causes of those manufactured associations. In this context, the authors of the NCEP update assume that the syndrome has a pathogenesis that can be discovered by studying genetics, molecular, biological, and cellular signaling:

> Moreover, a lack of understanding of the genetic and metabolic contributions to the causation of the syndrome stands in the way of developing new therapeutic approaches. The need exists, therefore, for additional basic and clinical research designed to better understand [the] pathophysiology [of metabolic syndrome] from the standpoint of genetics, molecular biology, and cellular signaling.[39]

The implication is that proof of a cause for metabolic syndrome will help improve its predictions about which groups will develop diseases, not help establish it as a disease in and of itself. Here, the effort to establish metabolic syndrome as a disease with a cause in a body seems to be combined with, or perhaps supplanted by, the need to use metabolic syndrome as an indicator of risk across populations.

Nonetheless, it was precisely these types of arguments about metabolic syndrome that encouraged the American Diabetes Association (ADA) and the European Association for the Study of Diabetes (EASD) to publish a critique of metabolic syndrome that called into question its legitimacy within biomedical science and its use within clinical practice.[40] While the ADA/EASD authors believe that metabolic syndrome may have been useful for educational purposes—to educate doctors about the clustering of risk factors for chronic disease—in the final analysis, metabolic syndrome has "taken on meaning and import greater than is justified by our current knowledge."[41] In the paper, the ADA/EASD advance a critique that lists the top eight reasons to be concerned about metabolic syndrome.[42] The authors also raise a new issue (at the time) about metabolic syndrome, namely, that because of the ways that some definitions of the syndrome use race to determine the statistical norms that construct obesity, these definitions identify different proportions of racial and ethnic minority groups as being at risk. For example, the prevalence of metabolic syndrome in Mexican Americans varied up to 24 percent between the World Health Organization (WHO) and NCEP definitions of the syndrome.[43]

Metabolic syndrome emerged through the technoscientific integration of molecularization and the risk factor paradigms, two social processes that were increasingly focused on understanding metabolism from a biomedical perspective. Accordingly, I argue that the extension of legitimate government authority over metabolic syndrome marks the emergence of a new discourse and technology of biopower. This emergence created a context in which the molecular processes of the body were used to construct risk-based syndromes of populations that social institutions such as professional biomedicine and the federal government could deploy to understand and improve metabolic health, especially among racially categorized groups. In the next chapter, I address questions of race and ethnicity in the emergence of metabolic syndrome.

CHAPTER THREE

The Scientific Racism of Metabolism

Since the National Cholesterol Education Program codified metabolic syndrome in 2001, different government agencies began publishing information about the syndrome on their Web sites. The following quotes represent what anyone who reads these Web sites would see about the relationship between metabolic syndrome, race, and ethnicity:

> Genetics (*ethnicity* and family history) and older age are other important underlying causes of metabolic syndrome.
>
> —NATIONAL HEART, LUNG, AND BLOOD INSTITUTE[1]

> Other causes of insulin resistance may include *ethnicity*; certain diseases; hormones; steroid use; some medications; older age; sleep problems, especially sleep apnea; and cigarette smoking.
>
> —NATIONAL INSTITUTE OF DIABETES AND DIGESTIVE AND KIDNEY DISORDERS (NIDDK)[2]

How is it possible for the federal government, via these communications to health consumers, to make the claims that ethnicity is (a) genetic and (b) a cause of metabolic syndrome? As a result of the implicit and explicit institutionalization of race in biomedical research, all racial and ethnic minority groups now are high-risk "special populations" that require institutionalized forms of metabolic examination, surveillance, and regulation. How, then, do concepts of race and ethnicity become institutionalized in the production of biomedical knowledge about metabolic syndrome?

One way to think about the puzzle that race presents for metabolic syndrome researchers is in terms of how to measure and interpret metabolic differences across individual bodies and population groups in ways that are consistent with prevailing cultural ideas about racial differences between bodies and populations. In the sections that follow, I interpret metabolic syndrome as a racial project, an unfolding representation of bodily and population difference that continually draws upon racial meanings to make sense of human metabolic differences. In some moments, the ways in which race informed metabolic syndrome was explicit, and in other moments, it seems to be implicitly woven into the everyday practice of doing biomedical research in the United States. In the broadest terms, the specific approaches to race in metabolic syndrome research were consistent with the broader cultural understanding of race as a marker of difference in American society. To examine this puzzle, I trace the production of racial meanings across three specific domains of metabolic syndrome science. First, I outline a brief history of scientific racism to establish a theoretical context for the racialization of metabolic syndrome. Then I show how early metabolic syndrome researchers' approaches to the study of human metabolism both explicitly and implicitly targeted bodies and populations based on prevailing racial categorizations that marked the metabolic processes of whites as the standard against which other groups would be compared. Second, I examine how metabolic syndrome researchers aimed to establish the causation of metabolic syndrome through conceptualizing race as a causal and genetic concept. Finally, I use the notion of "special populations" to show how race concepts are used to construct explanatory theories of "genetic admixture" in racial disparities research on metabolic syndrome.

A Brief Review of Scientific Racism

The coupling of race and metabolism within medicine, biology, and population genetics research is fueled by the new institutional knowledge-making practices that signal how technoscience shapes societies, particularly in the context of scientific racism. Scientific racism consists of discourses and practices that serve to explain and justify social inequalities as the natural outcome of hierarchically organized biological difference understood principally as racial difference. The traditional reading of scientific racism traces its emergence in the eighteenth and nineteenth centuries as a significant link between Western human sciences such as physical anthropology, comparative physiology, and biology and European imperialist projects such as colonialism and the eugenics movement.[3] The theoretical linkage between the use of skin color as a system for classifying and ranking human populations into groups called races and white-supremacist assumptions about the biological inferiority of nonwhite racial groups fueled public policy and made color-conscious scientific racism possible and potent. Critical race theories successfully challenged scientific racism by contesting the historical narratives and social practices of Western natural and social sciences.[4] One overarching project of critical race theory is dismantling the relationship between biology and race. As philosopher David Theo Goldberg argues, "race is the perfect medium for this collapsing of the social, the historical, into and upon the natural, of value into (claimed) fact, of 'seeing'—really conceiving—social conditions and relations, identities and subjectivities in natural terms."[5] If race constituted a major mechanism for naturalizing power, then identifying how race was not a natural biological category challenged the ostensible objectivity of science and therefore its centrality to political projects.

Scientific racism seemingly declined in the mid-twentieth century when its foundational assumption of racial essentialism was increasingly debunked in the aftermath of Nazi racial hygiene policies.[6] Scientific racism introduced racial essentialism—definitions of race based on presumed physiological, biological, and/or genetic difference—as a form of logic in Western science. Racial essentialism suggests that racial taxonomies reflect fixed and hierarchically ranked types of human populations that are classified based largely on skin color and visible physical features.[7] By the mid-twentieth century, the essentialist race concepts that had informed Nazi racial hygiene and genocide had become the object of international scientific scrutiny, impelling the production of the widely influential pronouncements by the United Nations Educational, Scientific and Cultural Organization (UNESCO) that commonsense notions of race lacked scientific basis. UNESCO argued that the term race "designates a group or population characterized by some concentrations, relative as to frequency and distribution, of hereditary particles (genes) or physical characters, which appear, fluctuate, and often disappear in the course of time by reason of geographic or cultural isolation."[8]

Critical race theorists challenged the scientific objectivity of race concepts, arguing that because scientific knowledge production was complicit with institutional structures of racial power, it was incapable of producing an objective science of race, but could at best produce racial narratives or "fictions."[9] This line of critique consisted of showing how the very categories of normal science that appeared to be value-neutral were in fact laden with racial meaning. Scientific knowledge did not just reflect racism—Western science was an active participant in constructing and maintaining racism. In other words, Western bioscience upheld racial projects but also itself depended on racial thinking. If science produced racial knowledge that justified these forms of racial hierarchy, then attacking the scientific basis of race, in particular knowledge produced by the social and natural sciences, constituted a potential remedy. Stated differently, because science generally, and scientific racism within it, was so central to racial rule, taking power away from science in defining race constituted a major political terrain of struggle. Normal science is seen as racist based on its history of collaboration with core social institutions such as the state, schools, the medical establishment, and insurance industries.[10] For example, critical race analyses have shown how eugenicists and statisticians collaborated to develop racist state policies and eugenics programs.[11]

Collectively, the pillars for critical race theorists' critiques of scientific racism involved working inside and outside of the paradigm of Western science, challenging it to become more empirically accurate and ideologically objective to the greatest extent possible. In essence, biological constructions of race as explanations for social inequalities were contested by challenging the veracity of a biological notion of race. Revealing the fallacy of a biological basis to race enabled critical race theorists to contest a range of associated practices, such as explaining racial disparities in health outcomes using biological criteria. Yet, refuting the biologically grounded notions of race did not mean that race disappeared from science. With biological conceptions of race now excised from scientific research on humans, scholars in a range of fields increasingly used social conceptions of race in their research and gave little credence to the discredited tenets of scientific racism. This is what happened in the burgeoning science of metabolic syndrome.

Sampling Normal Subjects

The physical examinations and laboratory tests that provided the early technological foundations of metabolic syndrome were developed using white European research subjects. Early studies of metabolic clustering are silent on issues of race. None of the samples that formed the evidentiary basis for early studies of metabolic syndrome contained any visible racial minorities, and there was no reference to whether the observed clustering of metabolic abnormalities varied across population groups classified according to race.[12] Thus, the white European body provided the empirical data for the construction of early ideas about metabolic syndrome. In other words, the metabolism of the European body became the norm against which other bodies would be compared, a standard practice in late-nineteenth-century and early-twentieth-century biochemistry and medicine.[13] As discussed in chapter 2, University of Marseilles physician Jean Vague is routinely cited as one of the primary originators of the metabolic syndrome concept because of his investigation of the potential causal relationships between obesity, heart disease, and diabetes. Vague defined his construct through a binary logic based on sex, and he believed that the more "masculine" the bodily form, the higher the likelihood of heart disease. His research on the index of masculine differentiation provides a good example of how race was overtly present by virtue of its covert absence. The ways in which Vague's key concept, the index of masculine differentiation, overlays the socially constructed category of sex over standardized anthropometric data provided a conceptual blueprint for how metabolic syndrome would overlay race categories over standardized biochemical and anthropometric data. Although the naked white skins of Vague's research subjects were published on the pages of the *Journal of Clinical Nutrition,* Vague and these early researchers never mention race.

In contrast to the covert racial meaning communicated through Vague's research, race became an organizing principle of the earliest American population-based research on metabolic health. Beginning in the 1940s, the federal government took on a new role in monitoring the metabolic health of the U.S. population. While epidemiological research, such as the Framingham study, provided the empirical basis for biomedical information about risk factors for heart disease in white populations, it was not until the 1980s that the U.S. government began to fund studies on non-European population groups specifically with regard to metabolic health problems. This more explicit focus on race, and the use of race to study the health of large populations, was in part a response to smaller community studies of diabetes, heart disease, and stroke that showed rates of metabolic disease on the rise in communities of color beginning in the 1960s and 1970s.[14] This new focus on race, and the new use of race to structure population health research, was also part of broader efforts to include racial and ethnic minorities in clinical and biomedical research.[15]

Population health studies were instrumental in the emergence of metabolic syndrome because they provided institutional mechanisms *by* which, and a discursive framework *through* which, conceptions about race and ethnicity could become attached to metabolic syndrome. Here, I highlight technical and racial frameworks of four of the earliest and most prominent of these federally funded studies, which were all modeled on the 1948 Framingham study. While they are broadly representative of numerous population health studies conducted all of over the United States, these four studies were significant theoretically and practically for three reasons: (1) they each included the specific examinations and laboratory tests necessary to classify metabolic syndrome; (2) they sampled and collected data from populations they explicitly conceptualized as racial; and (3) their data have been widely used to analyze metabolic syndrome *as* a racial construct.[16] In other words, they have been central institutional locations for the racial formation of metabolic syndrome.

The San Antonio Heart Study (1979–88) is important because it was the first major study after Framingham to measure all of the components of metabolic syndrome *and* to focus on a particular ethnonational group: Mexicans. It was a longitudinal cohort study that sampled five thousand residents of three areas of San Antonio, Texas. It was designed to identify factors beyond obesity that contribute to diabetes and cardiovascular risk in Mexican immigrants and Mexican Americans as compared to whites. These groups were sorted into low socioeconomic status (SES) "Mexican American," middle SES "Mexican and White," and high SES "White" research subjects.[17] By stratifying their study population by race and class in this way, the researchers made assumptions (for example, that whites cannot be poor and Mexican Americans cannot be wealthy) that impacted their study's findings. However, social class was not their primary object of investigation—"genetic admixture" was what they wanted to theorize. The physical examination collected data about "blood pressure, obesity, body fat distribution, [and] skin color, the latter to estimate percent Native American genetic admixture."[18] In their words, measurements of insulin resistance were compared to skin color to test the hypothesis that at any given level of adiposity Mexican Americans will be more insulin resistant than Anglos and that the insulin resistance in Mexican Americans is proportional to the degree of Native American ancestry.[19]

A second study, the Coronary Artery Risk Development in Young Adults Study (CARDIA), 1985–2006, was a prospective, longitudinal, multisite, cohort study that sampled 5,115 black and white men and women aged 18 to 30 in Birmingham, Alabama; Chicago, Illinois; and Minneapolis, Minnesota.[20] This study is significant because an explicit effort was made in the sampling strategy for CARDIA to achieve approximately balanced subgroups of race, gender, and education across age and geographic groups.[21] The CARDIA study has been widely used to evaluate the relationship between racial discrimination and blood pressure, as well as the relationships between dairy consumption and the insulin resistance syndrome.[22] An analysis of the list of publications on the study Web site shows that as of September 2014 at least thirty-eight studies have used CARDIA data to analyze metabolic syndrome, insulin resistance syndrome, or syndrome X.[23]

The Atherosclerosis Risk in Communities Study (ARIC), 1987–98, was a third population health study that was significant for the racial formation of metabolic syndrome because it was designed to "investigate the etiology and natural history of atherosclerosis, the etiology of clinical atherosclerotic diseases, and variation in cardiovascular risk factors, medical care, and disease by race, gender, and location."[24] ARIC was a prospective longitudinal study that sampled 15,792 individuals (aged 45 to 62) in Minneapolis, Minnesota; Washington County, Maryland; Forsyth County, North Carolina; and Jackson, Mississippi.[25] According to the study's Web site, the ARIC data have been used to publish at least thirty-one articles on metabolic syndrome, metabolic syndrome X, and multiple metabolic syndrome since the publication of its first wave of data in 1989.[26]

The fourth study is the Jackson Heart Study (JHS) (1987–2003), the largest prospective study ever of the "inherited (genetic) factors that affect high blood pressure, heart disease, strokes, diabetes and other important diseases in African Americans."[27] JHS began as one site of the aforementioned ARIC study. It sampled 6,500 African Americans, aged 35 to 84, living in Jackson, Mississippi.[28] According to the study description at the National Heart, Lung, and Blood Institute, the Jackson Heart Study included an extensive examination, including a questionnaire, physical assessments, and laboratory measurements of conventional and emerging risk factors that may be related to cardiovascular disease (CVD). The physical assessment of subjects in JHS includes height, weight, body size, blood pressure, electrocardiogram, ultrasound measurements of the heart and arteries in the neck, and lung function. The laboratory measurements collected from subjects includes cholesterol and other lipids, glucose, indicators related to clotting of the blood, among others. With these techniques, the Jackson investigators have been able to examine the "physiological relations between common disorders such as high blood pressure, obesity, and diabetes, and their influence on CVD."[29]

The population studies I highlighted in this section provided a techno-scientific means for inscribing metabolic syndrome with racial meanings. By linking race, population, and metabolism in specific ways, these studies, and the research products they generated, documented and explained racial group disparities in metabolic syndrome. These studies did not always generate analyses of metabolic syndrome and race that are grounded in biology and genomics (although they did make such groundings possible on a large scale); many researchers aimed to explain racial disparities in metabolic risk with reference to differential access to medical care and inequitably distributed exposure to stressful life circumstances such as interpersonal racism. However, as in the case of the San Antonio Heart Study, these population studies also served as a platform for the theory that racial group differences in metabolic risk could be explained by genetic admixture, as understood through the prism of race as biologic difference. Thus, racial disparities in metabolic risks are simultaneously interpreted as one outcome of living in racially stratified societies and the effect of genetically differentiated populations sorted into and known through race.

Is Race Really to Blame?

While these and other population health studies produced the biomedical surveillance data used to study metabolic syndrome, clinical researchers continued to use racial categorization in their research on metabolic syndrome at the level of individual bodies. In fact, the data that emerged out of race-based population studies provided a basis on which practicing physicians might understand their patients' metabolic health status differently depending on their apparent racial classification. From the epidemiological perspective that shaped government-funded race-based population studies, there was a need to understand whether and to what extent risks for metabolic health problems might differ across the main population groups of the nation. As will become apparent in this section, these questions about the *distribution* of metabolic health problems across racially categorized groups began to intersect with new theoretical questions about the *causes* of metabolic syndrome in racially coded bodies.

In addition to the four studies I have discussed, Stanford University endocrinologist Gerald Reaven's research constitutes a second useful site to examine how scientists conceptualized race and ethnicity in relation to the population dynamics and individual-level causes of metabolic syndrome. Along with Jean Vague, Reaven is revered as a second so-called founder of metabolic syndrome. In his 1988 Banting lecture, Reaven defined "syndrome X" as a series of six related variables that tend to occur in the same individual—resistance to insulin-stimulated glucose uptake, hyperglycemia, hyperinsulinemia, an increased plasma concentration of VLDL triglyceride, a decreased plasma concentration of HDL cholesterol, and high blood pressure.[30] Reaven did not note any explicit racial or ethnic distinctions in the syndrome X construct, nor in the etiological theories that he proposed to explain the relationships between insulin resistance, cholesterol, blood pressure, and heart disease risk.

However, a close examination of the clinical studies that formed the evidentiary basis for Reaven's theories about syndrome X reveal a pattern similar to Vague's ideas with respect to race. In his earlier research on insulin resistance during the 1970s, Reaven seems to have drawn upon mostly white European research subjects when he was part of a group of medical researchers at Stanford. Different members of the group (both including Reaven) published two studies in the *Journal of Clinical Investigation*: one in 1970 that tested a new technique for measuring insulin-mediated uptake and another in 1975 that demonstrated that this new method of measuring insulin resistance tends to identify subjects with diabetes.[31] The descriptions of the sample, which contains people with diagnosed diabetes and those without diabetes, are different in each paper in one exceptional way. In the 1970 paper, the authors describe how the diabetics in the sample were selected from their patient referral group, matched by weight, age, and percent adiposity with the normal control group. In this brief passage, they describe the sampling procedure for the normal population paper:

> Normal individuals were selected after interviews with a group of volunteers who had recently been discharged from a local minimum-security prison. Volunteers responded to a notice asking for assistance in a research project which would furnish their living expenses during a 2 week hospital stay.[32]

In the 1975 paper, the recently released inmates who likely participated in the study in order to get shelter are described simply and neatly as "healthy adult male volunteers." While neither study reveals nor refers to the race or ethnicity of its subjects, both the age and sex of each subject are noted in the printed tables. Without any evidence to the contrary, it is reasonable to assume that Reaven's subjects were predominantly white and/or that their race or ethnicity was immaterial to the analysis at hand. This is so given two facts: the overwhelming number of white Americans in 1970, and the fact that the mass incarceration of black men had yet to begin, so the prison population was composed mostly of whites. While sparse data exist on the racial distribution of prison inmates who volunteered for biomedical and behavioral research, participation in research projects entitled some prisoners to monetary and social benefits, to the exclusion of others. By failing to consider how race mattered in the formulation of his signature concept, Reaven excludes the possibility that race is in any way related to the problem of insulin resistance.

By 2000, racial health disparities had become a main intellectual and policy focus of federal health agencies. Also, by 2000, Reaven explicitly links race and the syndrome in his book *Silent Killer*. He states that people with genetic abnormalities, *people of non-European origin*, people with a family history of diabetes, heart attack, and hypertension, and people who eat poorly and exercise little are at a much greater risk for developing syndrome X.[33] To support this claim, Reaven cites three lines of evidence, two of which are drawn from research in which he participated that treat race and ethnicity as constructs that identify disease-relevant genetic differences between groups. For the first line of evidence, Reaven cites a 1985 study he coauthored that compared fifty-five Pima Indian men living near Phoenix with thirty-five Caucasian men living in California.[34] The investigators measured the levels of obesity, physical fitness, and insulin resistance in the two groups (who are not explicitly labeled as racial groups in any way) and used statistical techniques to determine the degree to which differences in their levels of obesity and physical fitness contributed to the variability of their insulin action. Reaven, now writing in 2000, claims that this 1985 study showed that "half of the variability of insulin action was due to lifestyle, the other half presumably to our genes. Of the 50 percent attributed to lifestyle, half was due to fitness, half to obesity."[35] Here, Reaven and his coauthors claim that half of the variability in insulin action was owing to population differences in genetics, which are measured by the criterion of race. This contention is based on the racial assumption that comparing Pima Indians and Europeans is equivalent to comparing underlying genetic differences between these population groups.

The second line of genetic evidence that Reaven cites also comes from research conducted on the same sample of Pima Indians.[36] This study compared levels of insulin resistance within Pima families to levels of insulin resistance across families and demonstrated, again, according to Reaven in 2000, that the clustering of insulin action is greater within families than it is across families. In effect, this claim constructs familial heritability and genetic susceptibility as the same biomedical phenomenon when it plays out within a tribal group with high rates of intermarriage. The third line of evidence that Reaven cites to substantiate the role he sees for genetics in causing syndrome X purportedly shows that American Indians, South Asian Indians, Japanese Americans, African Americans, Mexican Americans, Australian Aboriginals, and various Pacific Islander populations are more insulin resistant compared to people of European ancestry.[37] Reaven does not cite any studies after making these claims, but instead inserts a parenthetical statement that crystallizes his ideas about the causes of racial difference: the observed differences in insulin resistance reflect genetic differences between racial groups. Reaven and his collaborators argue that while it is *possible* that some racial groups might be more insulin resistant because of lifestyle habits and other factors, several studies *did take* all known group differences into account and concluded that differences in insulin resistance result from heritable genetic differences between groups.[38] Thus, the evidence that Reaven cites to support the claim that non-European bodies are more likely to develop syndrome X assumes that bodily differences in insulin resistance result from heritable genetic differences between racial groups that cannot be explained by other ostensibly nonracial factors. This form of essentialism positions race and ethnicity as heritable genetic structures that govern metabolic processes.

The New Special Populations

In addition to these efforts to link race, genetics, and the causality of metabolic syndrome, the uses of race in biomedical research on metabolic syndrome have expanded in new directions following the 2001 NCEP designation of metabolic syndrome as a secondary target of intervention. These expansions have taken place through the increasing interaction between new forms of biomedicine and government public-health research, both of which are focused on documenting, explaining, and intervening on group-based racial health disparities. Because of these converging forces, there is no lack of biomedical data about race and health in American biomedicine. The term "special population" is used specifically within government biomedicine to refer to pregnant women, children, racial and ethnic minorities, the elderly, and any other population group that is not white/European and male. The examination of racial health disparities constitutes one rationale for studying special populations that are sampled and targeted using constructions of race and ethnicity. People who are classified with metabolic syndrome or who think they have it are a new special population that is constructed out of and reproduces biological and genetic meanings of race. In this final section, I use the notion of special populations to show how race concepts are used to construct racially coded standards for biochemistry and physiology and explanatory theories of "genetic admixture" in research on metabolic syndrome.

Since 2001, scientists have increasingly raised questions about the use, measurement, and interpretation of metabolic syndrome when comparing different racial and ethnically defined populations. These new questions about the relationship between race and metabolic syndrome emerge from the enactment of several important technoscientific practices that target these special populations. First, since the World Health Organization recommended standardizing obesity measurements in different racial and ethnic groups first in 1997 and again in 2004, race and ethnicity have explicitly been used in the practice of validating group-specific empirical norms for one of the main physical examinations that comprise metabolic syndrome.[39] Because of the ways that some definitions of the syndrome use race to determine the statistical norm for obesity, these definitions classify different proportions of racial and ethnic minority groups with the syndrome. The argument for using race-based norms is that they improve the generalizability and validity of comparisons of disease risk across individuals within special populations. Statistical validity is determined with respect to the outcome—metabolic syndrome—by evaluating whether the syndrome successfully identifies all of the individuals who are at increased risk within special population groups. Thus, for example, the body mass index (BMI) for an individual who is classified "African American" would be statistically adjusted to account for the differential relationship between BMI and heart disease risk in African Americans as a population compared to other groups. These standardizations construct valid statistical norms against which racially and ethnically defined special populations can be meaningfully compared to one another.

In 2003, in their joint definition of the insulin resistance syndrome, the American Association of Clinical Endocrinologists and the American College of Endocrinology, two professional organizations of clinical and research endocrinologists, provided optional norms for obesity for different ethnic groups.[40] Three years later, in 2006, the International Diabetes Federation (IDF) incorporated racial and ethnic measurements of waist circumference because "there are clear differences across ethnic populations in the relationship between overall adiposity, abdominal obesity, and visceral fat accumulation."[41] The IDF elaborates a list of country-of-origin and ethnicity-specific values for waist circumference for "Europids," "South Asians," "Chinese," and "Japanese" populations. Several other groups do not yet have their own standardized values: "Ethnic South and Central Americans," "Sub-Saharan Africans," and "Eastern Mediterranean and Middle East." In the meantime, the authors advocate that the South and Central American ethnic groups should use "South Asian" values, and the "Arab populations" should use "European" values until "more specific data are available." The authors of the IDF study provide special instructions for applying these country- and ethnic-specific values in clinical and epidemiological research:

> It should be noted that the ethnic group-specific cut-points [norms] should be used for people of the same ethnic group, wherever they are found. Thus, the criteria recommended for Japan would also be used in expatriate Japanese communities, as would those for South Asian males and females regardless of place and country of residence.[42]

These recommendations imply that these norms should be used to compare "ethnic" populations that transcend "place and country of residence." These "ethnic" populations sound a lot like biological races, especially because constructs like place and country of residence profoundly shape ethnicity. Yet, this emphasis on ethnic populations obscures questions of race and assumptions about bodily differences that accompany race. To name these populations "ethnic groups" but then to sidestep the country-specific cultural dynamics that shape bodies' response to metabolic environmental exposures reveals that this use of ethnicity functions to deflate the potential criticism that these standardized norms are unabashedly racial and, at least potentially, racist. Since 2005, this focus on statistical normalization practices has informed a new body of biomedical research that explicitly investigates the implications of using metabolic syndrome to compare heart disease risk across different racially categorized groups.[43] Scholars in this emerging field of research have investigated racial and ethnic differences in the relationships between obesity and heart disease risk, body composition and metabolic risk factors, the power of triglycerides to predict insulin resistance, and the relationship between HDL cholesterol levels and CVD risk.[44]

African Americans, and theories of African American health, occupy a prominent place in special population research that links race and metabolic syndrome. A review article on metabolic syndrome in African Americans was published in the journal *Ethnicity and Disease* in 2003. All of the authors of this review article are members of the African-American Lipid and Cardiovascular Council (AALCC), a nonprofit health professional advisory group that is supported through an unrestricted educational grant from Bristol-Myers Squibb Company, and many of them have published widely on metabolic syndrome and African Americans.[45]

In the lead article, W. Dallas Hall and colleagues situate their review of metabolic syndrome and African Americans in the context of the epidemiological fact that African Americans have the highest overall CHD (coronary heart disease) mortality and out-of-hospital coronary death rates of any racial group in the United States. However, to explain the racial disparities in metabolic health between "Native Americans," "Mexican Americans," and "African Americans" *as compared to* "European Americans," the group features a "genetic admixture theory."[46] Theories of genetic admixture assume that individual-level risk for disease is related to shared genetic admixture with populations known to be susceptible to the disease. According to this theory, pre-1960s European Americans had historically had higher rates of diabetes than African Americans, Hispanics, and Native Americans, but increasing racial miscegenation that has occurred through decolonialization and racial desegregation explains the increasing rates of diabetes in these racial and ethnic minority groups.[47] The central assumption of this theory is that racial groups at an earlier moment were pure and segregated and it is their intermingling since the "discovery" of race that explains emergent trends in racial disparities in modern times. They argue that the degree of genetic admixture is related to the susceptibility of different racial groups to the risk factors that constitute metabolic syndrome. According to these authors,

> Whites of European origin appear to have greater predisposition to atherogenic dyslipidemia [high levels of LDL or bad cholesterol], whereas Blacks of African origin are more prone to HBP [high blood pressure], type 2 diabetes and obesity. Native Americans and Hispanics are less likely to develop HBP than Blacks, but appear particularly susceptible to type 2 diabetes. Of particular note is the considerable genetic admixture among Native Americans and Mexican Americans.[48]

As Duana Fullwiley makes clear in her analysis of how scientists use this logic of genomic admixture to make sense of Latinos' development of asthma, the new biotechnological tools used by these scientists mobilize old logics of racial difference in ways that affirm racial categorization and obscure the cultural imprint of the scientists on the knowledge-making process.[49] The focus on race within special populations research on metabolic syndrome has served as a location for the application of new technologies that map old racial categories onto groups defined by "genetic ancestry."[50] Genetic admixture analysis becomes a way of knowing racial identity as well as a strategy for determining metabolic risks. The focus on documenting racial differences in metabolic syndrome within biomedicine has accompanied the survival of theories of disease that attempt to link the biologies of racial groups to metabolic risk.

Metabolic syndrome folds group-based differences in the economic and political resources that are necessary for good metabolic health into a term that only references the biological processes in the body that create and use energy, a move that obscures the operation of institutionalized racism. Metabolic syndrome draws on and circulates racial meanings that construct race as a biological and genetic feature of bodies that can now be understood through technoscience. By grounding race in the body along with a predominantly biomedical understanding of metabolism (as opposed to a sociological or political one), these technoscientific practices have the unintended effect of obscuring the ways in which racialized social structures produce poor health for all people. These technoscientific practices remain linked to historical formations of scientific racism that explained racial inequalities as biological, natural, and immutable. Racial essentialism is central to the operation of scientific racism, a set of discourses and practices that served to explain and justify racial inequalities using the tools and authority of science. When analyzed in the specific context of racial health disparities, the use of essentialist notions of race to explain away racial inequality takes on special significance in the history of comparative racial biology and eugenics. One of the social implications of metabolic syndrome is that its practitioners do not address the ways in which it is both racialized and racializing, a remarkable omission given how central racial disparities in metabolic health have become to national debates on health injustice and the warnings about the return of scientific racisms through technoscience. This omission is especially problematic given the ways in which pharmaceutical corporations have both promoted and underwritten metabolic syndrome research and targeted particular racial and ethnic groups for the study and marketing of drugs.

CHAPTER FOUR

Killer Applications

The Racial Pharmacology of Prescription Drugs

Metabolic syndrome has emerged through an increasingly technoscientific and racial approach to understanding the risk of metabolic health problems. The risks associated with abnormal metabolic states among racial and ethnic groups were calculable, and these enumerations of biochemical and physiological processes had been the basis for biomedical intervention and treatment. In other words, your doctor ordered laboratory tests because she needed them to know if you needed help and, if so, how to help you. That process, at least with respect to cholesterol, has changed.

In November 2013, the American College of Cardiology and the American Heart Association published the findings of a four-year-long effort to reconsider clinical guidelines for the treatment of high cholesterol. Recall from chapter 2 that the cholesterol guidelines published in 2001 recommended metabolic syndrome as a secondary target of intervention. Their comprehensive review of available clinical and epidemiological evidence about cholesterol-lowering strategies yielded one startling recommendation that contradicted decades of scientific thought and practice: ignore the patient's cholesterol numbers. This was a huge surprise. The outcome of meetings like these had always been the same. Lower the standards. As with standards for other metabolic states such as blood pressure, obesity, and diabetes, the standards kept getting lower and lower, thus expanding the populations of people who are subject to biomedical surveillance and treatment regimes. The 2012 meeting was unique in one important respect: instead of meeting the empirical standard itself for high cholesterol, patients who are sorted into four risk categories should take as much statins as their bodies will allow in order to reduce their risk. As the report states, "the RCT [randomized clinical trials] evidence clearly shows that ASCVD [cardiovascular disease] events are reduced by using the maximum tolerated statin intensity in those groups shown to benefit."[1]

Now, I turn to prescription drugs and the study of drug metabolism in the racial science of metabolic syndrome. In the introduction, I mentioned that pharmaceutical corporations are interested in developing prescription drugs that could be sold to people who might be classified with metabolic syndrome and that this research has a new racial dimension. In chapter 3, I used the term "special populations" as a way of referring to the biomedical study of population groups who are not straight white men. This term has added significance in the context of drug research and development because just as biomedical research needed to include these nonwhite male groups, drug manufacturers are now required to study the safety and efficacy of prescription drugs in nonwhite populations. In this chapter, I build on this argument and analyze race and metabolic syndrome in biomedical research on drug metabolism and use of prescription drugs among African Americans.[2]

My analysis encompasses three distinctive arguments that connect race, metabolic syndrome, and prescription drugs: (1) racial pharmacology, the biomedical study of prescription drugs, their effects, and their metabolism in racially categorized bodies and populations, is an emerging site for the production of racial meaning;[3] (2) pharmaceutical companies and drug researchers use constructions of race to organize clinical trials, the development of killer applications, and the study of the genetics of drug metabolism; and (3) assumptions about genetic differences across racially categorized groups shape the racial pharmacology of killer applications.

To investigate these issues, I divide this chapter into three sections. In the first section, I develop the metaphor of killer applications to examine how prescription drugs operate in the politics of metabolism. As I will discuss later in the chapter, killer applications is a metaphor for novel combinations of human and non-human technologies that structure bodily practices in a wide range of social, commercial, and scientific contexts. The metaphor of killer applications is especially well suited for examining how prescription drugs operate in the politics of metabolism by transforming the ways that drug companies design, study, and market drugs for racially categorized groups. The analysis of killer applications I present illuminates how African Americans' metabolic processes have become the target for new forms of pharmaceutical capitalism in the United States. In the second and third sections, I compare the different racial meanings in the pharmacology of two killer applications:

atypical antipsychotics and statins.[4] Statins and atypical antipsychotics are prescribed for the treatment of schizophrenia and high cholesterol, respectively, and each has a unique relationship to metabolic syndrome. Yet, race and metabolic syndrome intersect differently in the pharmacology of antipsychotics and statins in ways that matter differently for African Americans. By comparing antipsychotics and statins along these dimensions, I document how race and metabolic syndrome intersect in the world of killer applications.

The Metaphor of Killer Applications

A biomedical–government–industry collaboration formed in 2002 focused on the relationships between diabetes and heart disease. On July 15, 2002, the Diabetes Mellitus Interagency Coordinating Committee held a meeting at the main campus of the National Institutes of Health in Bethesda, Maryland, to discuss "Macrovascular Disease and Diabetes: Translation Issues." The committee brought together representatives from the National Institutes of Health, the Centers for Disease Control, academic biomedicine, and the pharmaceutical industry to "determine the means and methods for translating the current scientific data from clinical trials and epidemiological studies to diabetes patients and the general public." The committee's responsibilities were to tell Americans about "an increased relative risk of cardiovascular disease (CVD) for those individuals who have been diagnosed with diabetes or pre-diabetes" and to propose ways that biomedicine, the federal government, and the pharmaceutical industry might work together to help in the translation effort. At this meeting, a pharmaceutical company representative encouraged a new line of pharmaceutical research on what he called "killer applications." He argued that so-called killer applications research on metabolic syndrome was needed because patients, such as those with metabolic syndrome, are taking multiple drugs for multiple health problems and a new killer application in this area might prevent the need for multiple drug regimens, or replace existing therapies by increasing efficacy or decreasing side effects. What is a killer application and what does it have to do with prescription drugs and metabolic syndrome?

The term "killer application" comes from multiple locations within the domain of technoscience. According to the *Oxford English Dictionary*, which added the term in 2001, the first public use of the term appears in *PC Week* in 1987: "Everybody has only one killer application. The secretary has a word processor. The manager has a spreadsheet."[5] Drawing on Donna Haraway's brief discussion of the term, I define it as a useful metaphor for novel hybrid combinations of human and nonhuman technologies that structure bodily practices in a wide range of social, commercial, and scientific contexts.[6] Technology companies of all stripes strive to develop killer applications to gain technological superiority and maintain market supremacy over their competitors. As Larry Downes and Chunka Mui explain, killer applications are a new good or service that "establishes an entirely new category and, by being first, dominates it, returning several hundred percent on the initial investment."[7] For example, killer applications structure the social practices of technology users, as was the case of the iPod. Within a few short years, the iPod revolutionized how people listen to music, interact with each other, and as a result of being the first of its kind, it still enjoys widespread popularity and brisk sales (at least in the form of the iPhone). In other words, killer applications enact the power to change modes of cultural and economic organization. Moreover, because of the myriad ways that killer applications impact how we interact with technologies of all kinds, including computer, communication, and biomedical technologies, they have the potential to change our bodies, collectivities, and societies in profound ways.

This metaphor of killer applications suits prescription drugs in four ways. First, prescription drugs fit the classic definition of killer applications because they are technoscientific commodities that combine nonhuman and human elements. The nonhuman element of prescription drugs consists of the drugs themselves. Prescription drugs are mostly synthetic chemical compounds and fillers that have been mass-produced in laboratories and factories. The human elements of prescription drugs as killer applications can be seen in the field of clinical pharmacology, the branch of biomedical science that studies the intended and unintended effects of drugs on the body. These human elements of prescription drugs consist of the relationships between medical professionals—typically doctors, who prescribe the drugs—and the patients who purchase and consume the drugs. The interaction of these nonhuman and human elements of prescription drugs qua killer applications represents a network of technoscientific and commercial relationships that fundamentally change human bodies. In this sense, prescription drugs are "applied" to bodies through a formalized process that involves drug companies, federal regulatory agencies, medical professionals, and consumers. In a sense, pharmaceutical research and development are entirely focused on manufacturing drugs that function like killer applications for any legitimate disease or disease in the making.

Second, because prescription drugs have revolutionized how American medicine treats illness and disease, the search for killer applications has taken on new cultural meaning within the pharmaceutical industry. As the industry has grown in scope and reach over the past half century, taking prescription drugs has become Americans' preferred practice for treating illness. When Americans get sick, they turn to their doctors and pharmacists for help—assuming that they have access to doctors and pharmacists and the financial means or insurance coverage to pay for them. If one is not feeling well, often the first question people ask is, "Are you taking anything?" When people get sick, all they need to do is ask their doctors for a prescription. Every day, Americans are bombarded with television and print direct-to-consumer advertising from the pharmaceutical industry that encourages them to ask their doctors about taking new drugs to treat what ails them. The killer applications metaphor helps us understand how a particular drug becomes a "blockbuster."

Third, risk management is the central tool for creating successful and profitable killer applications. The production of knowledge about risk was central to the emergence of metabolic syndrome and no less has risk influenced a biomedical and statistical approach to population-based drug development and research. For example, prescription drugs such as Lipitor acquire market supremacy by doing the best job of helping patients lower their risk of developing a particular condition, whereas other prescription drugs become successful because they do the best job of minimizing the risk of experiencing side effects from other drugs. The better a drug is at managing different kinds of risk, the more likely it will become a killer application. Recently, the term "comparative efficacy" has emerged in the debate over the future of the U.S. health-care system as a way to make it more cost-efficient.[8] Comparative efficacy refers to a process through which researchers compare possible treatments for a health problem in order to determine which treatment, or combinations of treatments, is most likely to be effective at treating the problem.

Fourth, because of the rise of metabolic health problems in the American population, the pharmaceutical industry has a special interest in killer applications that target them. The health problems encapsulated by metabolic syndrome currently account for one-fifth of all health-care spending in the United States and much of that money is spent on prescription drugs. The U.S. pharmaceutical industry has been among the most profitable industries for years, in large part owing to prescription drugs that are sold to the millions of individuals who suffer from metabolic conditions such as heart disease and high cholesterol. In 2004, four of the top ten

most-dispensed drugs treated hypertension or high cholesterol, two central pillars of metabolic syndrome.[9] By 2013, six of the nineteen biggest
drug blockbusters of all time were compounds that treat metabolic health
problems, with Lipitor at the top of the list at $13.69 *billion* in sales.[10]
Interestingly, three of the nineteen best sellers are atypical antipsychotics
(#7, Abilify; #15, Seroquel; and #19, Zyprexa). With the appearance of
metabolic syndrome, the pharmaceutical industry has at least sixty million new potential customers and some new challenges, some of which
are centered on race. The central challenge that race poses for killer applications is this: if race is a socially constructed category, then how can
drug researchers use race to identify which bodies and populations need
particular killer applications, or particular doses of killer applications?

In recent years, numerous scholars have raised a series of questions
about how drug researchers use race to develop, study, and market prescription drugs.[11] Many of these new questions about race in pharmaceutical research have emerged in response to the controversy over BiDil,
the first drug approved by the FDA in June 2005 for specific use among
African Americans. BiDil (isorbide dinitrate/hydralazine hydrochloride) is
not a new chemical compound—rather, it is a new patented combination
of two existing generic drugs. As these scholars have identified, one of
the central questions in the BiDil case was how industry researchers used
racial categories to frame their investigation of whether subpopulations
varied with respect to drug response and metabolism. Sociologist Troy
Duster cautions biomedical researchers, especially those associated with
drug companies, against committing the fallacy of reification with regard
to race—the tendency to assume that our categories of thought coincide
with the obdurate character of the empirical world.[12] Duster questions
how NitroMed, the producer of BiDil, presented statistical information
about racial disparities in congestive heart failure in ways that mis-
represented the extent and etiology of racial disparities between African
Americans and whites. This misrepresentation in the case of BiDil reifies
race by arguing that different racial groups have "genetically sufficiently
distinctive features . . . which are used to explain health disparities between racially categorized populations."[13] These kinds of essentialist discourses about race have established an important historical justification
for scientific racism.

Philosopher Lisa Gannett asks whether federally created and self-
reported race, ethnicity, and ancestry are, in fact, good proxies for genetic
similarities in drug metabolism.[14] She argues that the debate about the

use of racial categories in clinical trials and pharmacological research has often been framed in terms of realist versus social-constructionist theories of race. The realist theory of race claims that our racial classifying practices identify things in nature, and that race is therefore a scientific and objective category. The social-constructionist theory of race asserts that race is not a genuine natural category but an invention of racialist/racists societies, hence subjective. Gannett steps through this debate by noting that this framing of the epistemological status of race assumes that boundaries can be inserted between "the social and scientific, the cultural and natural, and what is objective and subjective."[15] According to her, a priori racial taxonomies of human groups, such as those used in pharmacological research, do not exist independently of social classifying practices in specific research contexts.

To analyze these emerging practices, Gannett advances a pragmatist epistemological framework that includes an ethical analysis of the use of group categories in pharmacogenomics research. What this means is that scholars need to ask questions about the potential harms enacted upon racially categorized groups if the very categories designed to track and rectify the effects of systemic racism become biologized through their incorporation in scientific research, clinical practice, and the marketing of pharmaceuticals. Rather, attention to health-related group differences need not perpetuate the racist history that has seen some communities shoulder a disproportionate share of the burdens associated with biomedical research while reaping fewer of the benefits.

These developments are part of what I refer to as racial pharmacology, or the biomedical study of prescription drugs, their effects, and their metabolism in racially categorized bodies and populations. Clinical pharmacology is the branch of biomedicine that studies the intended and unintended effects of drugs on the body. Clinical pharmacology can be understood as comprising three interconnected fields of study: pharmacokinetics, pharmacodynamics, and pharmacogenomics. Pharmacokinetics studies the biological processes by which bodies absorb, distribute, metabolize, and excrete drugs. Pharmacodynamics studies the effects of drugs on bodies, the mechanisms of drug action, and the relationships between drug concentration and effect. Pharmacogenomics investigates the relationships between drug pharmacokinetics, pharmacodynamics, and genetics. Each of these fields of clinical pharmacology has a racial structure that shapes the research and development of killer applications.

In the following sections, I compare and contrast the racial meanings that emerge from the racial pharmacology of two killer applications—antipsychotics and statins—that are both associated with metabolic syndrome, yet in different ways. The first case focuses on atypical antipsychotics, a class of prescription drugs that doctors prescribe to treat schizophrenia but that produce the negative side effects of obesity, high cholesterol, and high blood sugar—side effects that comprise metabolic syndrome.[16] In the case of antipsychotics, researchers use metabolic syndrome as a discourse about the undesirable side effects of killer applications such as antipsychotics. African Americans have been disproportionately diagnosed with schizophrenia, have been underrepresented in clinical trials for schizophrenia-related drugs, are overprescribed antipsychotic injection therapies, and are said to differ genetically from other racial and ethnic groups in terms of antipsychotic metabolism. Because the treatments for schizophrenia have become racialized, the diagnostic category of schizophrenia also becomes racialized through the deployment of killer applications.

The second case focuses on statins, a class of drugs that physicians prescribe to treat dyslipidemias, which are fundamental to the construction of metabolic syndrome. In the case of statins, researchers use metabolic syndrome as a discourse about potentially broader uses of existing killer applications such as statins. African Americans are constructed as having differential rates of high cholesterol, are the primary subjects in new clinical trials for statins, are underprescribed the most effective statin therapies, and are said to differ genetically from other groups in terms of statin metabolism. In order to justify race-based treatments, high cholesterol is being framed as a new racial disparity that requires new studies in drug efficacy and safety.

Specifically, I compare these two killer applications across four key dimensions of racial pharmacology. First, I ask how scientists use race to study the underlying health conditions that are related to each potential killer application. In the case of antipsychotics, the underlying health condition is schizophrenia and in the case of statins, the underlying condition is high cholesterol. The racial dynamics of each of these conditions is linked to how race is taken up in killer applications research. Second, given the treatment of race in the study of the underlying condition, I ask how race is used to organize clinical trials for these killer applications. How well are African Americans represented in clinical research on these drugs and what are the implications of this participation? Third, I ask how race is used to organize the routes of administration and consumption of these killer applications. Are African Americans underprescribed or overprescribed particular killer applications? How might ideas about race shape these practices? Fourth, I ask how race is deployed to frame questions about group differences in African Americans' drug metabolism. How do assumptions about genetic meanings of racial difference shape the science of drug metabolism? By comparing antipsychotics and statins along these four dimensions, I document how race and metabolic syndrome intersect in the study of killer applications.

Atypical Antipsychotics and African Americans with Schizophrenia

Metabolic syndrome has become a way of measuring whether racially categorized bodies require different modes of atypical antipsychotic therapy because of the risks of weight gain and diabetes associated with their consumption. Analyzing the side effects of atypicals using metabolic syndrome has become a new focus of schizophrenia drug research. A diagnosis of schizophrenia made by trained mental health professionals should be a prerequisite for prescribing any antipsychotic medicine. Yet, like metabolic syndrome, the diagnostic category "schizophrenia" must be interrogated in relationship to the knowledge-making practices that have produced psychiatric illness taxonomies.

There are three prevailing theoretical interpretations of what mental illnesses are: constructionist, biological, and professional. Social-constructionist models of mental illness argue that illness categories, such as schizophrenia as constructed in the Diagnostic and Statistical Manual of Mental Disorders (DSM), represent cultural definitions applied to different types of bodies and behaviors, and whose contours and meanings change over time.[17] Prior to the 1980 publication of the DSM-I, a biological view of schizophrenia was widely accepted within mainstream American psychiatry. The biological view of mental illness maintains that psychiatric symptoms, and the taxonomies they are used to construct, reflect undetected biochemical and genetic processes in the body. The DSM was supposed to standardize mental illnesses and establish a scientifically informed professional practice organized around their diagnosis and treatment. Thus, the professional psychiatric model understands mental illnesses such as schizophrenia as "a spectrum of syndromes that are classified by clusters of symptoms and behaviors considered clinically meaningful in terms of course, outcome, and response to treatment."[18] According to the Diagnostic and Statistical Manual of Mental Disorders-IV (DSM-IV), an individual can be classified with schizophrenia if he/she reports the following:

a disturbance lasting at least 6 months and . . . including two or
more of the five symptom groups: (a) delusions; (b) hallucinations;
(c) severely disorganized speech; (d) grossly disorganized or catatonic
behavior, or (e) negative symptoms (e.g. affective flattening, alogia/
poverty of speech, and avolition/inability to initiate and persist with
goal-directed activities) with social and occupational functioning).[19]

Based on this categorical definition and professional view of mental illness,
schizophrenia is itself a syndrome that defines 1 percent of the American
population—roughly four million people.[20] More recently, a hybrid of
the biological and professional conceptions have been ascendant as the
diagnostic categories cataloged in the DSM are now understood through
a biological and genomic prism. Much of the current National Institute of
Mental Health research funding apparatus is geared toward developing
this hybrid approach to mental illness.

Since the rise of professional psychiatry in the nineteenth century, psychiatrists have assumed, asserted, and eventually accepted that African
Americans were more likely to suffer from schizophrenia.[21] One reason for
this prevailing view about African Americans and schizophrenia had to do
with the statistical methods that were widely used to produce knowledge
about population rates of mental illness. Prior to the emergence of the
DSM in 1980 as the diagnostic tool for counting cases of schizophrenia,
the treated-case method was the preferred method for psychiatric epidemiology, which only counted subjects who received inpatient treatment in
mental health institutions.[22] During this period, African Americans made
up a disproportionately high portion of those individuals who were institutionalized for schizophrenia, especially during the era of mass institutionalization of the mentally ill between 1900 and 1940.[23] Because
psychiatrists assumed that African Americans were more likely to have
schizophrenia, they institutionalized them at higher rates. African Americans were overrepresented among institutionalized populations; therefore, the treated-case method produced inflated estimates of group illness,
which reaffirmed racist theories of African Americans' mental inferiority.
Accordingly, as Jonathan Metzl points out, psychiatrists in the 1960s
also began to redefine definitions of schizophrenia around the bodies and
behaviors of African American men.[24] By the 1990s, community-based
studies, such as the Epidemiologic Catchment Area (ECA) study and the
National Comorbidity Survey (NCS), were established as the accepted
method for determining population rates of mental illness.[25] These population studies and others showed that African Americans are still more
likely to receive diagnoses of schizophrenia and report higher levels of

psychotic symptoms compared to whites.[26] Despite the fact that racist ideas about the prevalence of schizophrenia among African Americans had been partially challenged, the emerging field of racial pharmacology created new problems and new questions.

Beginning in the 1950s, based on the prevailing biological view of psychiatric illness, psychiatrists began to treat schizophrenia using powerful new medications called antipsychotics. The first generation, or so-called typical antipsychotics, instantly became the killer applications for the pharmacological treatment of schizophrenia and other psychoses.[27] Beginning in the 1980s, scholars began to study group differences in access to and use of atypicals. In the 1980s and 1990s, researchers found that psychiatrists prescribed typicals at higher rates and in higher doses to African Americans in both inpatient and outpatient psychiatric settings.[28]

In the 1990s, pharmaceutical companies began to develop a second generation of antipsychotics called "atypical" that were supposed to avoid extrapyramidal side effects. The six atypicals and their year of FDA approval are Clozaril (clozapine) in 1990, Risperdal (risperdone) in 1994, Zyprexa (olanzapine) in 1996, Seroquel (quetiapine) in 1997, Geodon (ziprasidone) in 2001, and Abilify (ariprazole) in 2003. Since their introduction in the 1990s, atypical antipsychotics have become the new killer applications for the treatment of schizophrenia and have become a major source of profit for pharmaceutical companies, costing as much as ten times more than typical antipsychotics.[29] In 1999, the status of atypicals as killer applications was affirmed when professional psychiatric treatment guidelines were modified to name atypical antipsychotics as "first-line drug therapy" in the treatment of schizophrenia.[30]

Atypicals continue to dominate the antipsychotics market, yet they too create serious side effects. In November 2003, a biomedical–government–industry collaboration led by the American Diabetes Association and the American Psychiatric Association (APA) met to discuss the causes and consequences of the observed correlations between atypical drug therapy and diabetes.[31] The conference, titled "Consensus Development Conference on Antipsychotic Drugs and Obesity and Diabetes," brought together an industry–academy–government collaboration to address the question.[32] A consensus view emerged that psychiatrists should closely monitor their patients' metabolic biomarkers because of the known metabolic side effects of atypicals.

It is in this context that two noted schizophrenia researchers, Wayne Fenton and Mark Chavez, claim that metabolic syndrome is emerging as the tardive dyskinesia of the second-generation antipsychotics.[33] In 2004, the FDA issued a warning that atypical antipsychotics increased the risk of developing diabetes on its "news show"—FDA *Patient Safety News*.[34] The FDA asked drug manufacturers of atypicals to add new warnings to their labels informing patients of these risks; it also recommended that patients taking atypicals have their blood sugar levels checked periodically. Also in 2004, a group of psychiatrists issued specific recommendations for monitoring the metabolic health of people diagnosed with schizophrenia.[35]

The 2003, the APA/ADA group also urged researchers to determine whether the risks of therapy are increased in certain ethnic groups (e.g., African Americans).[36] There has been a general lack of scientific information about the safety and efficacy of antipsychotics in African Americans. For instance, one study found that African Americans may be more likely to gain weight while taking atypicals.[37] Researchers have documented basic patterns between African Americans' access to and use of atypicals compared to other racial and ethnic groups. African Americans categorized with schizophrenia are *more likely* to receive atypicals via injection as opposed to pill therapy.[38] Several groups of scholars have documented that African Americans with schizophrenia are *less likely* to receive atypicals than white patients with schizophrenia.[39] A 2001 Surgeon General report titled "Mental Health: Culture, Race, and Ethnicity" included a listing of the representation of racial groups in twenty-five randomized controlled trials for the treatment of schizophrenia that took place between 1986 and 1996. While sixteen of the twenty-five studies collected and reported data on the race and/or ethnicity of their research subjects, none of these conducted (and then reported) analyses by race or ethnicity. The remaining nine studies did not collect information on the race or ethnicity of research subjects, and did not conduct analyses by race or ethnicity.[40]

The 2001 Surgeon General's report also advanced a biological explanation of the different pharmacokinetics (the processes by which bodies absorb, distribute, metabolize, and excrete drugs) of antipsychotics in African Americans: more of them are "slow metabolizers." Citing a 1977 study, a 1982 study, and a 1998 study, the report claims that "a greater percentage of African Americans than whites metabolize some antidepressants and antipsychotic medications slowly and might be more sensitive than whites."[41] The report offers two contrasting arguments about the clinical significance of race in the pharmacological treatment of schizophrenia. On the one hand, it argues that "*biological similarities* between African Americans and whites are such that effective medications are suitable for treating mental illness in both groups." On the other hand, it cites recent studies that suggest that "African Americans and white Americans *sometimes* have different *dosage* needs."[42] These seemingly contradictory arguments position race both as immaterial to antipsychotic metabolism and central to it. What might explain this racial ambiguity?

The Surgeon General's report mentions the P450 system as a possible genetic source of these observed racial pharmacokinetic differences among schizophrenic patients taking atypicals. Mary Relling and colleagues found racial differences between "American black and white subjects" in debrisoquin hydroxylase (P450IID6) activity, a biochemical and genetic process implicated in drug metabolism.[43] James Walkup and colleagues explain the slow metabolizer theory of racial group difference in the P450 system as follows:

> Drug metabolism is mediated through the cytochrome P450 micosomal enzyme system. Small numbers of individuals lack the P450 microsomal enzyme and, consequently, are "poor metabolizers." Their plasma levels tend to be high. Recent studies have identified a larger group who are genotypically heterogeneous "slow metabolizers." Recent estimates suggest that the prevalence of slow metabolizers of antipsychotic medications is higher among African Americans and Asian groups than whites.[44]

In their conclusion, Relling et al. suggest, it is logically possible that *unmeasured physical differences* in pharmacokinetics might be responsible for differences in the metabolism of antipsychotics between white and African American or Hispanic individuals.[45] Here, the racial ambiguity is made clear: race represents the unmeasured physical differences between groups that explain why they appear to metabolize the drugs differently.

Statins and African Americans with High Cholesterol

Cholesterol researchers, and statin manufacturers, use metabolic syndrome and race as ways to identify which bodies and populations are most likely to benefit from statin therapy. Statins have become the killer application for the treatment of cholesterol problems (dyslipidemias), a key component of metabolic syndrome, and have become the world's most prescribed drug class. Statins are a class of cholesterol-manipulating drugs that were first approved for sale in the United States in 1986 and went on the market in 1987.[46] The first statin approved by the FDA in 1987, lovastatin, introduced the practice of treating "surrogates" into the FDA drug approval process and private drug research and development. A surrogate is a biological marker that is transformed into a statistical stand-in for a hypothesized disease process or outcome. So, LDL cholesterol is a surrogate for the development and growth of plaque in the arteries and in the heart.[47] LDL, or low-density lipoprotein, is the so-called bad cholesterol that has long been considered a risk factor for heart disease and stroke. Rather than needing to demonstrate that lovastatin reduced the incidence of heart attacks or strokes in a long-term prospective clinical trial, the investigators needed only to show that the drug agent affected the surrogate in expected (and desirable) ways in order to gain FDA approval.[48] The pharmacological treatment of cholesterol as a means of reducing heart disease risk is an outgrowth of the so-called lipid hypothesis, namely, that lowering LDL cholesterol alone will stop or slow the development of heart disease. As of 2013, seven statins are available in the United States for the treatment of dyslipidemia.[49]

Formal clinical guidelines for the pharmacological management of cholesterol identify statins that are used to determine the adequacy and equitability of patient care. As discussed in chapter 2, the 2001 guidelines issued by the National Cholesterol Education Program stood as the expert recommendations for the management of cholesterol until late 2013.[50] Given the stringent nature of these recommendations, many individuals with dyslipidemia will not be able to achieve optimal LDL cholesterol levels without pharmacological therapies, even with adequate exercise and changes in dietary practices.[51] Crestor (rosuvastatin) is one of the newest statins made by AstraZeneca that lowers LDL cholesterol and raises HDL cholesterol. Just one year after its FDA approval in 2003, fifteen million individuals filled prescriptions for Crestor, spending $908 million. Crestor is prescribed to people who have high LDL cholesterol and low HDL cholesterol, two biochemical criteria of the syndrome. In August 2008, AstraZeneca began mass-marketing Crestor after a new clinical finding that, along with diet and exercise, it can slow the progression of atherosclerosis.

Are the makers of Crestor, a new statin, framing the racial pharmacology of statins in order to be able to market them to racially categorized groups? In 2003, the pharmaceutical giant AstraZeneca started the Galaxy Program studies, which, according to the company's Web site, is a "large, comprehensive, long-term and evolving research initiative designed to address unanswered questions in statin research and to investigate the impact of Crestor on cardiovascular risk reduction and patient outcomes."[52] The Galaxy Program funded three six-week randomized, controlled, open-label, multicenter clinical trials that were designed to evaluate the safety and efficacy of Crestor in populations with hyperlipidemia—populations that were sampled using racial and ethnic categories.[53]

To organize these trials, AstraZeneca followed the FDA's guidelines for including racially categorized groups in clinical trials. For example, the African American Rosuvastatin Investigation of Efficacy and Safety (AIRES) trial is a randomized, controlled, open-label, multicenter trial designed to evaluate the efficacy of Crestor in 774 African American subjects by comparing it to Lipitor.[54] This study evaluated the achievement of cholesterol treatment goals in a sample of African Americans and non-Hispanic whites. The ARIES sample consisted of non-Hispanic whites and African Americans, although the methods of determining the subjects' ethnicities are omitted from the description of the study's methodology.[55] The study's cholesterol treatment goals were based on the 2001 National Cholesterol Education Program (NCEP) Adult Treatment Panel III definitions for dyslipidemia, the same risk category criteria that are included in metabolic syndrome.

The hypothesis for the study was that racial and ethnic differences in statin metabolism and management may partially account for the excess risk of mortality experienced by racial and ethnic minority groups. The investigators found that body mass index (BMI), total cholesterol, and LDL cholesterol were higher in African American subjects (which confers higher disease risk), but HDL and triglycerides biomarkers were better (which confers lower disease risk). African Americans were significantly less likely to meet ATP III LDL-C treatment goals within each risk category and overall. They were less likely to be taking statins than whites (75.7 percent versus 70.6 percent) and less likely to be taking high-efficacy statins (54.8 percent versus 45.6 percent).[56] Even among subjects taking statins and high-efficacy statins, fewer African Americans reached ATP-III targets for LDL-C.

According to the researchers, the explanations for the alleged ethnic disparity in cholesterol management were "not immediately apparent."[57] The disparity cannot be explained by differences in dyslipidemia diagnoses or access to health care because both the African Americans and the non-Hispanic whites in the sample were recruited because they were already receiving treatment for dyslipidemia. Fewer African American subjects were taking statins and they received treatment from lipid specialists less frequently. Therefore, less aggressive treatment on the part of treating physicians may partially explain the disparity. However, the statistical association between ethnicity and cholesterol goal achievement remained after controlling for these differences.

Group differences in rates of drug compliance may also account for these differences in cholesterol management. The authors cite three studies published since 2000 that suggest that African Americans are less compliant with statin drug therapy than are non-Hispanic whites.[58] The authors conclude that "It is likely that the explanation for lower frequencies of treatment goal achievement among African American patients for lipids and other therapies is multifactorial."[59] They cite socioeconomic status, educational level, and type of medical and prescription drug coverage as the multiple other factors affecting goal achievement, but their data did not permit the analysis of these other factors.

Clark and colleagues cited evidence that cholesterol responses to lifestyle modifications and drug therapies are "generally similar" in African American and non-Hispanic white subjects.[60] However, three of the four studies that they cite analyzed samples that consisted only of African Americans, including the ARIES trial, and thus could not have compared racial and ethnic groups.[61] In their conclusion, they cite these same four studies again and state that data from clinical trials of lipid-lowering drug therapies suggest that African American and non-Hispanic white subjects exhibit similar physiological responses.[62] Because the effects of lifestyle intervention and drug therapy do not vary across African American and nonwhite Hispanic populations, they hypothesize that the lower rates of cholesterol management among African Americans must result from (a) less aggressive management by treating physicians, (b) suboptimal compliance by African American patients, or (c) some combination of these factors.

In a 2007 article titled "Metabolic Syndrome in African Americans: Implications for Preventing Coronary Heart Disease," Luther T. Clark and Fadi El-Atat review several therapeutic approaches to metabolic syndrome in African Americans. While the magnitude of LDL-C reduction with statins appears to be similar in blacks and whites, the authors cite data from the Antihypertensive and Lipid Lowering Treatment to Prevent Heart Attack Trial (ALLHAT-LLT) study that showed that statin therapy lowered the risk of death from coronary heart disease and nonfatal heart attacks more in black than in nonblack subjects, but did not decrease the mortality gap overall between the two groups.[63]

In 2008, Dr. Karol E. Watson, an associate professor at the Geffen School of Medicine at UCLA and director of the UCLA Center for Cholesterol and Lipid Management, published a review article in the *Journal of the National Medical Association* titled "Cardiovascular Risk Reduction among African Americans: A Call to Action."[64] As a member of the speaker's bureau for AstraZeneca, Merck, Schering-Plough, and Sanofi Aventis, Watson reviews evidence that the major risk factors for cardiovascular disease require special study and intervention in the African American population. She argues that while data on racial and ethnic differences in response to lipid-lowering drugs are limited, two studies have shown that statins are not as effective at lowering African Americans' LDL levels compared to European Americans.[65]

Toward the end of her review article, Dr. Watson has a subsection titled "Race-Based Therapeutics," which is in quotation marks. The section begins:

> The development and use of so-called "Race-based therapeutics" remains controversial. Results of some clinical trials indicate that racial/ethnic differences in vascular function may have implications for the treatment of CVD risk factors.[66]

Here, she makes the argument that African Americans may have a different endothelial response to ACE (angiotensin-converting-enzyme) inhibition than European Americans because

> Individual response to the pleiotropic effects of statins, such as their beneficial effects on renal function independent of lipid lowering, *may also be affected by race.* In one study of short-term rosuvastatin treatment, estimated glomerular filtration rate increased by >3-fold in African American patients compared with the overall study population.[67]

To substantiate this second claim, she cites one study.[68] She then argues that "the fact that African Americans and European Americans appear to exhibit differences in endothelial and vessel wall response suggests that alternative strategies may be needed to customize therapy appropriately for patients of different races/ethnicities."[69] For Watson, the case of BiDil serves as an exemplar of these alternative strategies for race-based therapeutics. She concludes this section by rejoining that BiDil may work equally well in other racial/ethnic groups and that more research is needed in this area.[70]

The racial pharmacology of killer applications, the ways in which race is mobilized in the pharmaceutical industry, is a central feature of the politics of metabolism. Three interrelated developments comprise the central relationships in racial pharmacology. First, as illustrated in the case of statins, pharmaceutical companies are interested in creating racially circumscribed markets for their killer applications. Because the pharmaceutical industry is part of a capitalist system that exploits human health as a commodity, constructions of racially categorized risk groups are easily adopted into drug research and marketing strategies that seek to profit from presumed forms of racial difference that are thought to have a meaningful relationship to individual-level differences in drug metabolism. Second, following the 2005 FDA guidelines on the use of racial classifications in clinical trials, clinicians use race to study group differences in these metabolic processes that may be related to variability in drug responses.[71] Third, as I have suggested through both cases, drug researchers are concerned that pharmacokinetic, pharmacodynamic, and pharmacogenomic differences between individuals map onto racial categorizations that organize groups of individuals.

Pharmaceutical drugs as killer applications represented one set of biotechnologies that are related to the causes and treatments of metabolic syndrome. Another critically important set of biotechnologies related to the causes and treatments of metabolic syndrome are foods. Because metabolic syndrome encompasses multiple biochemical and physiological risk factors for disease, it has been correlated with a growing list of biochemicals that make up the foods that, in calculable ways, influence the levels of those same risk factors: sugar, fat, and salt. Given the widespread accusations levied against sugar as the toxic cause of America's metabolic health crisis, it is ironic that, for centuries, sugar has been constructed and used as a medicine.[72] The next chapter takes up this question of sugar and its relationship to the metabolism of African Americans and society.

CHAPTER FIVE

Sugar Stained with Blood

African Americans, Sugar, and Modern Agriculture

> There is not one barrel of sugar comes to Europe which is not stained with blood.
>
> —ANDREW VAN HOOK, *Sugar: Its Production, Technology, and Uses*

Within rural African American communities, the term "sugar" has multiple meanings, one of which is that "sugar" is a disease otherwise known as diabetes.[1] Designed to challenge and supplant cultural knowledge of diabetes, such as that represented by the use of the term "sugar" by African Americans, the application of technoscience to questions of food, nutrition, and health is a core feature of the politics of metabolism. People living with diabetes have to self-regulate their blood sugar—this is accomplished through balancing the sugars they consume relative to the insulin they need to absorb those sugars into the cells in their bodies. Sugar provides the energy cells need to function; insulin is a hormone produced by the pancreas that enables the absorption of sugar into cells. When I started on an insulin pump in 1995, I had to learn a new way to quantify and regulate the relationship between the food I ate and the insulin doses I administered: carbohydrate counting.

Carbohydrate counting involves adding up the total grams of carbohydrates in any food (minus the grams of fiber) and dividing this number by a number specific to my body—say, 12. The result of this simple math equation is the number of units of insulin that I need to give myself to compensate for the carbohydrates I was about to eat. I would add up the number of grams of total carbohydrates per serving, multiply by the number of servings, subtract the grams of fiber, and then divide by 12.

According to the training I received from my diabetes nurse educator and endocrinologist, it did not matter which carbohydrates I ate. The dominant practice at the time suggested that I was to treat all complex and simple carbohydrates equally—glucose, fructose, lactose, maltose, or any other kind of sugar—because they had identical effects on my blood sugar levels. In some ways, this new practice of carbohydrate counting made my life as a person with diabetes much easier than it had been under the old dietary regime. I could not eat whatever I wanted (that wouldn't have been wise for other reasons), but at least as far as my blood sugar was concerned, I only needed to worry about one nutrient. Carbohydrate counting placed special emphasis on sugar as the principal target of diabetes management; control sugar, control diabetes. Issues of fats, cholesterol, and sodium were not on the radar for me as a person living with diabetes.

The old regime, started in 1950, was based on "food exchanges," measurements of quantities and weights of foods that corresponded, roughly speaking, to food groups.[2] My goal was to eat meals that had a balance of items from different food groups: three starch exchanges, two protein exchanges, and one fat exchange. It was a nonintuitive system that required learning, memorizing, and successfully interpreting exchange values and the corresponding weights and measurements of foods contained within each group. The exchange system was also a less precise and calculable system, leaving open possibilities for blood sugars that were too high or too low. Still, the system had its advantages, the most important of which is that the exchange system framed each meal as a food experience that had to demonstrate balance and equity on the plate. Although I might not need to give more or less insulin because of the fats or proteins I was planning on eating, I at least needed to consider them as part of the equation.

Despite its strengths, I rejected this old system of food exchanges for a new life as one of Donna Haraway's cyborgs, opting to regulate blood sugar through the use of insulin pump technology and carbohydrate counting.[3] These shifts in how I coordinated meals and insulin regimens occurred all the while I was eating highly processed foods, fast food, and pretty much whatever I wanted to eat as a college sophomore. Food exchange books enumerated the exchanges for these industrial foods as well. Growing up in a working-class African American family in the 1980s, I happily packed Little Debby snack cakes into my school lunches, ate microwavable French fries and milk shakes, and drank Coke just like everyone I knew. Just because I had been diagnosed with diabetes did not mean that I had to stop eating at McDonald's; it just meant that I now needed to give myself insulin so that I could eat it. Modern nutrition science and biomedical technology seemed to work well for me by allowing me to eat what I thought was real American food.

Jane Dixon describes the ways in which nutrition science complexes have shaped the production of "nutricentric" people whose lives are "ruled by biomarkers."[4] A nutrition science complex encompasses "temporally and spatially specific laboratories, observation and enumeration technologies, corporate and government sponsors, and a professional corps adept at enrolling discursive devices to manage producer–consumer relations through creating the 'nutricentric' citizen."[5] Dixon argues that a process of nutritionalization, "the co-option of nutrition science to extract surplus value and authority relations from food," underlies the formation of agricultural capitalism and its relationship to human metabolism.[6]

It is not possible to provide a critical interpretation of the politics of metabolism without recognizing the synergistic relationships between food regimes and human metabolism. A food regime is a "rule-governed structure of production and consumption of food on a world scale."[7] According to Phillip McMichael, food regime analysis "prioritises the ways in which forms of capital accumulation in agriculture constitute global power arrangements, as expressed through patterns of circulation of food."[8] Drawing on intellectual frameworks in Marxist thought, world systems theory, and historical and comparative sociology, food regime analysis positions food and agriculture as historical systems of power linked to global dynamics of capitalism, technoscience, ecology, and culture.

According to John Bellamy Foster, the concept of metabolism (*Stoffwechsel* in German) was first used as early as 1815 and was used by German physiologists to describe material exchanges within the body—specifically, the exchanges involved in processes of respiration. Beginning in the 1840s, Foster explains that European scientists such as Justus von Liebig, Julius Robert Mayer, Theodor Schwann, and John Tyndall vigorously debated the multiple meanings and embodiments of the metabolism concept and, through this process, established biochemistry and quantitative ecology as sciences.[9] These sciences were organized around a new conceptual focus on energy in the effort to understand and manipulate life. Presently, the concept of metabolism is a key concept in systems theories signaling the processes of biochemical exchange, regulation, and growth that define the relationship between material organisms and their environments. Scientists did not develop these ideas about metabolism in the nascent field of biomedicine; rather, conceptions of metabolism were deployed in the application of science to questions in capitalist agriculture about soil commodification and productivity. Yet, the conceptualization of the materiality of food nutrients at the molecular level synchronizes perfectly with the parallel shifts within biomedicine and pharmacology.

Scientific debates about the concepts of metabolism in agriculture drew the attention of Karl Marx, who, as Foster points out, had been incorporating materialist analyses of political economy *and* nature into his scholarship since he wrote his 1841 dissertation on the philosopher Epicurus. Whereas metabolism was used in biological theories to describe the processes that generate and regulate the energies within the human body, Marx used the concept of metabolism in his social theories to describe the processes by which human labor generates and regulates energies trapped within nature. Marx used the concept of metabolism in two ways: first, to refer to the cyclical processes by which people transform nature and themselves through the labor process; and second, in a broader sense, "to describe the complex, dynamic, interdependent set of needs and relations brought into being and constantly reproduced in alienated form under capitalism, and the question of human freedom it raised."[10] For Marx, industrialized agricultural capitalism creates a "metabolic rift" that redefines and disturbs the historical relationships between people and the earth on which human life depends. In *Capital,* he explains this metabolic rift:

> Large landed property reduces the agricultural population to an ever decreasing minimum and confronts it with an ever growing industrial population crammed together in large towns; in this way it produces conditions that provoke an irreparable rift in the interdependent processes of social metabolism, a metabolism prescribed by the natural laws of life itself . . . Large scale industry and industrially produced agriculture have the same effect. If they are originally distinguished by the fact that the former lays waste and ruins labour-power and thus the natural power of man, whereas the latter does the same to the natural power of the soil, they link up together in the later course of development, since the industrial system applied to agriculture also enervates the workers there, while industry and trade for their part provide agriculture with the means of exhausting the soil.[11]

Through material resource extraction and wage systems, capitalist modes of exploitation not only alienate workers from themselves, the process of labor, and other workers (the alienation of labor), they also alienate people from the earth (the alienation of nature).

Justus von Liebig, the progenitor of agricultural biochemistry whose ideas shaped Marx's theory of social metabolism, also was the founder of nutrition as a biochemical science in the late 1840s.[12] During this time and through the 1870s, colonial and imperial states quickly seized upon the new science of nutrition as a way to increase national power, security, and influence in ongoing transnational struggles over natural resources, land, and labor power.[13] In other words, the science of food—and, through the insertion of that science into capitalism, food itself—became a great technology of state power.

Science-based education for diabetes self-management has emerged with the consolidation of a whole scientific system organized around nutrition and metabolic health. How does this system construct and explain the relationships between African Americans, metabolic syndrome, and sugar? African Americans occupy a unique position as the producers and consumers of sugar within capitalist food regimes. At the same time, the nutrition sciences that accompany and facilitate agricultural capitalism have focused substantial attention on African Americans as a group because of their risks for metabolic syndrome. These scientific discourses about African Americans' food cultures often take place absent a contextualized discussion about how technoscientific and economic shifts in the capitalist production of food have impacted human metabolism. In the next sections, I explore how sugar figures into African American biopolitics and the nutrition science complex organized around metabolic syndrome.

Sugar and African American Biopolitics

It was none other than Christopher Columbus himself who brought sugar to the Americas in 1493. His father-in-law owned a sugar plantation on Madeira and so Christopher, ever the opportunist, brought sugar cane plants back to the island of "Hispaniola" on his first return trip hoping to establish a new sugar industry in the world he had discovered. Although the sugar cane he had planted thrived, the people who tended to the crop "often sickened and died."[14] By the middle of the sixteenth century, sugar would become one of the most valuable commodities grown in the New World, made profitable by millions of African slaves forced to work in sugar colonies and on sugar plantations throughout South, Central, and North America. The United States, Portugal, Spain, Italy, Belgium, the Netherlands, England, France—these national beneficiaries of the commodification, mass production, and consumption of sugar established a monumental structure for racial oppression whose shadow still lingers today.

Racially organized systems of sugar *production* were central to the growth of the slave trade, colonialism, and racialized capitalism in the United States, and hence they feature prominently in structures of African American oppression.[15] Sugar was a major cash crop in the slaveholding American South:[16]

> It has been reckoned that during the centuries when sugar-slavery flourished, some ten million Africans were carried across the Atlantic, mainly to man the sugar plantations . . . Sugar did not create Negro slavery . . . but without sugar the whole dark episode in human history, causing untold suffering and leaving consequences which curse the world today, would not have taken place.[17]

The insertion of sugar into global industrialized processing systems resulted in a staggering increase in sugar production from 8 million tons in 1900 to 70 million tons in 1970 to a projected total of 182 million tons in May 2014.[18] Over the course of its colonial and industrial history, sugar production has increased more rapidly than any other agricultural commodity.

Racially organized systems of sugar *consumption* are also central to the creation and maintenance of the racial subordination of African Americans. Neoliberal capitalism demands that multinational food corporations increase their profitability through the mechanism of market growth and closure made possible through technoscientific innovations.[19] This process is comparable to that of multinational pharmaceutical corporations that also increase their profitability through expanding markets (by disease mongering) and creating killer applications. The foods that are associated with the development of metabolic health problems have long been the objects of scientific study, government regulation, and corporate commodification within global agribusiness. The historical period during which metabolic syndrome emerged also brought substantive changes to the ways that food was produced, marketed, and distributed, which in turn shape the distribution of metabolic health problems.[20]

The sugar that was available to African Americans during slavery would have been in the form of molasses (made from sorghum) or sugar cane, both of which were grown throughout the South. During slavery, sugar was a luxury commodity to which many slaves did not have access.[21] Fannie Clemmons, a former slave interviewed as part of the WPA slave narrative project, recounts: "And sugar—we did not know about that. We always used sugar from molasses. I don't think sugar been in session long. If it had I did not get it."[22]

In the antebellum period, sugar became a more prominent feature of African Americans' diets. According to an 1895–96 U.S. Department of Agriculture (USDA) study mediated through Booker T. Washington's Tuskegee Institute, molasses was one of the staples of the Negro diet, along with salt pork, cornmeal, milk, and wheat flour:

> The molasses from sorghum is generally preferred to that from cane. The molasses is made on the farms by a very primitive process. This consists in passing the cane between rollers to squeeze out the juice, and boiling the latter in open pans, which are set on furnaces roughly built of stone and clay.[23]

African Americans favored highly sugared foods and drink for their taste and

> out of biological and physiological necessity to adapt to long hours of work in the plantation fields. Sugar provided a source of quick energy crucial to otherwise poorly fed slave workers, and it is believed that fat and salt contributed to the ability to sustain long hours in the fields.[24]

African Americans' foodways (the patterns of what they eat) are often blamed for their high rates of metabolic health problems. The claim is that their diet is high in fat, sugar, salt, and cholesterol and therefore they have higher rates of obesity, diabetes, and heart disease than other racial and ethnic groups. Thus, the cultural lifestyles of African Americans are blamed for their poor health. "Lifestyle" refers to individuals' and groups' patterns of daily life in terms of diet, exercise, and nutrition.[25] One review of African Americans' dietary practices makes a popular argument about culture:

> Many historical and cultural factors influence the current dietary intake and food choices of African Americans. The dietary habits, food choices, and cooking methods of African Americans evolved from a long history of slavery, persecution, and segregation. Slaves who were brought to the USA combined their West African cooking methods with British, Spanish, and Native American (American Indian) techniques with whatever foods were available to produce a distinctive African American cuisine called "soul food."[26]

Formations of African American food cultures are routinely linked back to slavery without any discussion of the intervening years in which their food cultures changed inside capitalist food regimes.

Sugar, African Americans, and Metabolic Syndrome in the Nutrition Science Complex

What empirical evidence supports the theory that sugar consumption changes a body so that it meets metabolic syndrome criteria? I hesitate to say that "sugar causes metabolic syndrome." Here's why: scientists cannot prove this claim as a fact. The phrase "causes metabolic syndrome" requires a few epistemological caveats. First, because metabolic syndrome is a syndrome and not a disease, it cannot have a cause and remain a syndrome in name only. If scientists identified a common and universal set of biochemical, genetic, and/or environmental conditions that would generate metabolic syndrome in every body, the syndrome would no longer be identical with itself—it would be a disease. Second, there are so many competing definitions for what constitutes metabolic syndrome in a body that identifying a common set of factors that apply across all of its current definitions seems unlikely. Despite major institutional efforts to harmonize the metabolic syndrome concept in theory, in practice, it is what researchers say it is.[27] Third, the set of biomarkers that comprise metabolic syndrome each has its own biological processes and pathways in the body and is impacted by different sets of biochemical, genetic, and environmental conditions. By definition, the multifactorial nature of metabolic syndrome belies efforts to identify a common cause—human metabolism is a highly complex and contingent process. Fourth, the gold-standard form of evidence that would provide definitive proof of a causal relationship between sugar consumption and metabolic syndrome would have to come from a randomized controlled clinical trial in which one group (the control group) ate no sugars for a period of time and the other group ate a lot of sugars (the experimental group). Such an experiment might also have the control group avoid eating any other food nutrients that might be related to metabolic syndrome such as cholesterol or fats. Such a study would be unethical because the researchers would knowingly expose the experimental group to conditions (eating lots of sugar) that they know are harmful to metabolic health. I doubt that these caveats, which all concern how scientists produce and validate claims about metabolic syndrome, are what matter most for people when it comes to their metabolic health.

As with every other scientific question, the details of this research are inconclusive (scientists don't know everything) and contingent (the details and contexts matter). However, several independent studies, meta-analyses, and scientific reviews have provided compelling and conclusive evidence that the consumption of sugar, especially fructose, generates unhealthy metabolic states that are codified into metabolic syndrome.[28] Sugar consumption initiates metabolic processes that change insulin production, blood sugar, and weight (obviously) but also lead to changes in cholesterol levels and inflammation (not so obviously).

The consumption of sugars has a huge impact on metabolic states. When a nondiabetic person consumes sugar, the brain informs the pancreas to secrete insulin so that the insulin can seek out the sugar, bind with it (as well as other molecules like hemoglobin and oxygen), and transport it through cellular walls throughout the body. When a person consumes a lot of sugar on a regular basis, the pancreas has to work overtime, secreting more insulin than it expects to—this leads to a metabolic state called hyperinsulinemia (high levels of insulin in the blood stream). Having too much insulin in the blood leads to a metabolic state called insulin resistance (described in chapter 2), in which the insulin the pancreas secretes becomes less effective in its task of binding with sugar. This process is pronounced in overweight people—their bodies have a difficult time producing enough effective insulin to compensate for the excess sugars in their bloodstream.

Sugar consumption also increases the number of calories that a body has at its disposal for running the all of the body's processes and actions. If a person does not use or burn more calories than he or she consumes, those surplus calories are converted into and stored as fatty tissues. Eating too much sugar leads to weight gain. A second parallel process unfolds in the liver when a nondiabetic person consumes the sugar fructose. Fructose is absorbed into the small intestine and then first metabolized in the liver, largely without the role of insulin.[29] The liver converts fructose into glucose (one of its component sugars) and the fatty acids triglycerides and LDL cholesterol (both of which are biomarkers of metabolic syndrome). High levels of triglycerides in liver cells also contribute to insulin resistance, liver disease, and hypertension. Let me keep it simple. "Added sugars" refers to sugars that food corporations and food preparers add to food that was not there to begin with. If there is one food practice people could change that would have a big, direct, and lasting impact on their metabolic health, it would be to severely limit or eliminate any "added sugars" in their diets.

How do nutrition scientists frame race and ethnicity when they are talking about African Americans and sugar metabolism? The opening sentences for nearly every population health research article that addresses questions of African Americans and metabolic health sing the same sad song of race, risk, and burden:

> African Americans carry significantly higher risk for cardiovascular disease than non-Hispanic whites in the United States today, and this is associated with higher rates of obesity, diabetes, hypertension, and ESRD [end-stage renal disease].[30]

> The increased prevalence of noninsulin-dependent diabetes mellitus (NIDDM) in some ethnic groups and the potential causes are of considerable interest. Compared with whites, rates of diabetes are 70–100% higher in black men and women in the 20–74 year age range.[31]

> The African American (AA) population has been shown to be at a higher risk for both obesity and the metabolic syndrome than are Caucasians.[32]

Why? African Americans consume more added sugars in their diets than other racial and ethnic groups.[33] Individualist arguments are frequently mobilized to justify and explain racial health inequalities. Biomedical individualism provides an important ideological framework for biomedical research and theories about diet-related diseases in contemporary food regimes. Liberal individualism is a political philosophy that emphasizes the rational actions of autonomous individuals in a free-market economic system. The proliferation of techniques of biological examination and surveillance and the construction of risk-based syndromes becomes comprehensible only within an ideological framework that views health as an individual moral responsibility.[34] According to Nancy Krieger and George Davey Smith, biomedical individualism features "a tendency to study decontextualized biology and genes and to reduce problems of population health to a matter of individual lifestyles plus faulty genes."[35] Biomedical individualism shapes biomedical discourses about African Americans' metabolic health in two main ways. First, the "bad" or "risky" choices of individuals are responsible for causing health problems. If people choose to eat unhealthy foods, or they smoke, or they don't exercise, they deserve the negative effects of those choices: "They had it coming." Second, the remedies for poor health are also located in individuals, through the widespread application of risk-reduction models for behavioral change. In these public-health models, individuals are encouraged to eat in healthier ways, not smoke, and exercise because these activities can reduce disease risks. Because African Americans shoulder a disproportionate burden of disease under the perspective advanced through biomedical individualism, they must also accept personal responsibility for their actions.

The substantive focus on individual choice and diet-related disease elides much-needed attention on the role of food corporations in shaping metabolic states. Individuals must make healthier choices because corporations and the government will not intervene to transform the current food regime. If people develop illness because of the foods they eat, they are responsible, regardless of the tactics, deceptions, and practices of food corporations and insufficient government regulations. Despite the fact that the great majority of processed American food products are unhealthy (the system of choices), food corporations lobby to ensure that no single product is implicated in disease or becomes the object of increased regulatory scrutiny.[36] The idea is that because any individual food can be incorporated into a well-balanced diet, no particular food should be regulated within the food market. In other words, food markets should operate freely so that consumers have the right to consume any products they wish, even harmful ones. Free capitalist markets are the source of all solutions to social inequalities and any attempts to remedy racial inequalities in health by tinkering with the market will be met with stiff resistance.[37]

African Americans' food choices are not the only subject of explanations of racial health inequalities. Nutrition scientists claim that African Americans metabolize the added sugars they consume differently than other racial and ethnic groups because of genetic differences. One argument is that African Americans produce more insulin (hyperinsulinemia) in response to sugar than whites.[38] Another is that African Americans are 3.5 times more likely to be "sweet likers" (people who seem to have a physiological and genetic preference for sweet-tasting foods) than other racial groups.[39]

African Americans (along with other nonwhite racial groups) are also theorized to have a so-called thrifty gene. In the 1960s, University of Michigan geneticist Dr. James Neel advanced a thrifty gene hypothesis—the idea that the expression of a thrifty gene varied between first- and third-world populations with progressing conditions of modernization, and that this variation in genotypic expression would confer a metabolic advantage in hunter-gatherer societies and preindustrial agricultural societies and a metabolic disadvantage in societies experiencing rapid

Westernization, specifically, the replacement of low-fat and nutrient-dense indigenous foods with high-energy foods brought on through industrial food processing. This theory was presented in a major National Institutes of Health report on diabetes in 1995:

> Neel suggested that populations exposed to periodic famines, *which occur in Africa,* would through natural selection increase the frequency of certain genetic trait(s), "thrifty genes," which would protect against starvation during times of famine. These genes would allow for efficient energy conservation and fat storage during times of abundance. In circumstances of relative plenty, as in the United States in the absence of feast and famine cycles, these genes would become disadvantageous, predisposing to the development of obesity and an increased frequency of NIDDM [type 2 diabetes]. The higher rates of diabetes and obesity in African Americans and urban Africans compared with black Africans in traditional environments is consistent with this hypothesis. An active search for NIDDM genes is being conducted.[40]

The thrifty gene hypothesis is still very much considered a viable explanation for racial disparities in metabolic health and has been given new life by a surge in genetic research, despite the fact that there is no genetic evidence whatsoever for the gene itself.[41]

However, the extent to which individual-level choices or genetics shape group-based metabolic health problems is an empirical question, one that has been addressed within the rich history of social-science research on the fundamental causes of disease that highlights the role of group-based differences in social power and exposure to health-promoting and/or disease-causing social conditions. The ways in which race and social class intersect to limit access to healthy foods and increase access to unhealthy foods reflect not only the practices of transnational food corporations but the broader structures of neoliberal capitalism. This research has barely penetrated national consciousness, public-policy debates, or the nutrition science complex.

As with pharmaceutical drugs, technoscientific innovation in food science leads to "breakthroughs" that can be mobilized by corporate and government actors to achieve market expansion and consolidate political power. Foucault argued that agricultural innovation is one of the central features of the emergence of biopower—the power over food represents the extension of disciplinary and regulatory power over life itself. The significance of food biopolitics is also apparent in stark contrast to the deployment of killer applications and the cultural power that prescription drugs have over people's metabolic lives. Indeed, the economic interests of agricultural and pharmaceutical corporations operate in our very bodies and shape the politics of metabolism in ways that go beyond posing food and drugs as disconnected political issues. As we have seen in this chapter, this could not be further from the truth.

Metabolic Insurrection

The NIH RePORTER, a searchable database of National Institutes of Health–funded research projects, lists 18,848 studies between 2001 and 2014 that are relevant to "metabolic syndrome" at a cost of $8,140,486,609.[1] As we saw in the Introduction, many thousands of research articles have been published on metabolic syndrome since 1989. How many academic and professional conference presentations featured the syndrome? What concrete benefits did all those research projects, journal articles, and conference presentations deliver the people who live and die within the politics of metabolism?

At a recent visit to the endocrinologist, I asked my nurse practitioner what she thought of metabolic syndrome. Her blank response suggested to me that she had never heard of it, and it wasn't the first time that one of my own medical providers expressed ignorance of it. Although the syndrome has garnered an ICD-9-CM diagnosis code since 2001 (277.7), the practice of using the code to diagnose actual patients is, to quote CDC analyst Earl Ford in 2005, "rarer than a blue moon."[2] In his analysis of the National Ambulatory Medical Care Survey and the National Hospital Discharge Survey, Ford found that in 2002, sixteen out of 327,254 medical records listed the 277.7 code; in 2003, only eleven records did so. Since that one analysis published in 2005, no one has replicated this analysis to see whether doctors are literally diagnosing metabolic syndrome in their patient populations. Only one article evaluates its actual use in clinical practice. Of the thousands of research articles published on metabolic syndrome, none directly analyzes what practicing doctors themselves think about the syndrome. I did not find *one* published study conducted in the United States that asks people who might be categorized with metabolic syndrome what they think about the idea. In this real sense, metabolic syndrome is an entirely theoretical construct. The flexibility, portability, and mobility of a discourse of metabolic syndrome across the American biomedical landscape are its most impressive features, and perhaps its only material features. Metabolic syndrome is a biopolitical paper tiger.

In 1956, the same year that Jean Vague began publishing articles on what would later be called metabolic syndrome, Chairman Mao Zedong called the United States a paper tiger—the United States seemed powerful in theory, but in reality it was powerless. In his essay "The Resistance to Theory," literary theorist Paul de Man decried those in the literary community who had a problem with the pretentious incursions of something called literary theory. Those people who resist literary theory, he wrote, are themselves producing theory through their resistance to theory. So, what's the problem with theory, then?

> It is a recurrent strategy of any anxiety to defuse what it considers threatening by magnification or minimization, by attributing to it claims to power of which it is bound to fall short. If a cat is called a tiger it can easily be dismissed as a paper tiger; the question remains however why one was so scared of the cat in the first place.[3]

If metabolic syndrome is a biopolitical paper tiger because doctors are not actively diagnosing people with it and the people themselves don't know about it, why be concerned about its emergence in American biomedicine? If it is just a fetish, a textual flash in the pan of a fully biomedicalized corporate science, can't we just ignore it and move on with the real, material health issues facing people?

Metabolic syndrome is a discursive symptom of a gaping metabolic rift in the United States (and globally). It is a clear sign that the social relationships between people, their food systems, their healing systems, and the political and intellectual institutions that are supposed to be working in and for their best interests (i.e., governments and universities) are fundamentally severed. People who suffer from being overweight, who are beginning to experience the deleterious consequences of diabetes, who have had a stroke or heart attack, are living in the chasm created by the metabolic rift in America. Do these people (myself included) need another study of metabolic syndrome to alert them to this rift? What kind of evidence could such a study (or twenty thousand more studies) provide that would be more compelling, more persuasive, more conclusive than our own collective, embodied experiences as people living and dying within the politics of metabolism?

Critical social theories raise questions about the conditions that are subjecting groups of people to injustice and oppression and open up possibilities for their mutual survival, escape, and resistance. This book has raised many questions about metabolic syndrome and its emergence with the nexus of the state, scientific, and capitalist structures of biopower. Most centrally, I have been concerned with interrogating the structure of meanings that link metabolic syndrome to concepts of race and ethnicity and the institutional practices that create and sustain racism. Metabolic syndrome serves as a site for the reproduction of race because its users draw on and circulate racial meanings that construct race as an immutable, fixed, biological, and genetic feature of bodies. The syndrome serves as a discursive mechanism for racism because scientists use it in ways that obscure the biopolitical relationship between racism and health in the United States. When it comes to race and racism, metabolic syndrome makes the metabolic rift, and the racial health injustices that define it, seem to be completely natural. Racial and ethnic minority groups have higher rates of metabolic health problems because that's natural for them. It's in their genes, their cultures, their choices. But this could not be further from the truth.

Technoscience provides a way to understand how the increasingly technological and scientific aspects of metabolic syndrome come together to shape its racial meanings. In the political context of biomedicalization, molecular processes and genetic differences provide the authoritative scientific explanations for racial differences in health; racism has nothing to do with it. By using this new concept of metabolic syndrome, researchers are positioned to argue that racial groups have unequal rates of metabolic health problems because metabolic processes are fundamentally different across racially categorized bodies. Yet, metabolic syndrome also became a new technoscientific object about which researchers could author genetic conceptions of race that serve to explain racial inequalities in metabolic health. While all groups have to live and die within the politics of metabolism, African Americans shoulder a disproportionate burden of metabolic health problems. The sociological and biological reasons for this burden of disease are complex and multifactorial—there is not just one theory that answers every question about health injustice. However, a critically important insight that this book offers to ongoing efforts to explain the racial health injustices that

African Americans experience is that technoscientific practices that construct racial meaning still matter.

Challenging Color-Blind Scientific Racism in Bioscience

Bioscientific theories of race still matter in the early twenty-first century. As discussed in chapters 1 and 3, critical race theories have recognized the centrality of science and medicine to the construction of racial concepts and meanings that in turn influence the practices of social institutions.[4] Critical race theorists in the twentieth century thought they had debunked scientific racism, a set of color-conscious scientific practices that looked to bodies themselves as the primary signifier of race and then mobilized visible bodily differences as justification for racial subordination.[5] Race was written on the skin, which served as the linkage between the raced body and the social hierarchies that became attached to race. Scientific racism functioned in a color-conscious context that visibly identified racial populations and subordinated them via color-conscious policies. Although racial meanings within science were not always constructed through comparisons of visible external differences, skin color has remained the central signifier of embodied racial difference, particularly in the American context.[6] This phenotypical racism based on skin color continues to structure social inequalities across and within racially categorized populations.[7]

Biological theories of race based on color-coded classifications of bodies have been largely discredited.[8] Yet, it is also apparent that discrediting biological theories of race did not necessarily mean that racism itself, or well-intentioned attempts to redefine race in the language of biology and genomics, would disappear.[9] Grounding race as inherent to the biology of human beings is an epistemological precondition to what has been alarmingly called the return of scientific racism. Science and technology studies scholars have warned that the resurgence of the study of racial difference and inequality in bioscience marks "the biological reification," "biological rewriting," and "genetic reinscription" of race.[10] These terms connote the sense that the contemporary biosciences reproduce ideas of race as a materially real object that can and should be discovered through the investigation of bodily materials quite literally beneath the skin.

The conceptual decoupling of race *as* skin color and the emergence of new formations of race *as* genes and biochemicals within the biosciences has taken place in a broader racial shift from color-conscious to color-blind forms of racial oppression.[11] As a critical social theory, the task of critical race theory thus lies in unsettling the assumptions, scholarship, and social practices that make racism invisible and discrimination possible and justifiable. One important contribution of critical race theory has been investigating the workings of color blindness as a new racial formation.[12] *Not* seeing color constitutes the new ideology dedicated to creating a socially just society.

Color blindness operates as an ideology whose effect is to obscure the material practices of racism and racial structure.[13] In reality, color blindness upholds racial hierarchy by diverting political and scholarly attention from the racialized social structures that protect white privilege.[14] The logic of color blindness is that because race, and therefore racism, no longer exists, the subordinate status of people of color becomes a problem of innate individual failings, poor choices and ignorance, and biological susceptibility, not globally institutionalized racism.[15] The attention to color blindness also highlights the relationship between social distance and power—the multicultural vision of America promotes racial inclusion, yet practices of racial exclusion determine who gains access to the substantive rights of citizenship.[16]

Color-blind racism is a new system of power that conceals racial hierarchies and structural inequalities by sanctioning the use of race.[17] Analyses of color-blind racism focus on structural racial inequalities, namely, the continued marshaling of empirical evidence to "prove" that racial disparities persist despite color-blind racism's claims that they have been eliminated.[18] One outcome of this emphasis in critical race theory has been the emergence of sophisticated theoretical analyses of how color blindness produces (as opposed to fails to challenge or merely accommodates) structural inequalities and the ideologies that justify them. For example, Lani Guinier and Gerald Torres argue that, despite legal frameworks that identify color blindness as foundational for democracy, the law uses color-blind practices such as redistricting to produce racially disparate outcomes.[19] Similarly, David Theo Goldberg contends that not only do modern states fail to uphold the ideal of equal justice, but they use discourses of color blindness or racial neutrality in order to function as racial states.[20] Similar efforts have been devoted to reading common social practices that reproduce color-blind racism, such as everyday strategies that whites use to justify racial inequalities and maintain white privilege while avoiding seeing race.[21] Despite these contributions, efforts to dismantle racism can arrive prematurely at the belief that identifying the "fiction" of race constitutes the end point of analysis.[22] This leads to one erroneous assumption, namely, that the persisting criticisms of racism for being color-conscious will be equally effective against forms of color-blind racism.

A second emphasis in critical race theory investigates how Western conceptions of modernity rely on the logic of racial distinction.[23] This attention to racial logic has refocused attention on binary thinking as foundational to Western institutions. Racial categories provided the discursive tools through which European societies could organize themselves as ordered, rational, and objective. In particular, the Western rationality that imposed colonial orders on so-called primitive worlds constitutes the same practice of racialization that was deployed to construct and enforce modern state policies. These fundamental features of modern science, its objectivity and rationality, gain meaning only in the context of race. The process of achieving rational order consists of reducing individuality by aggregating individuals into population categories that can be manipulated.[24] Modern states and scientists created racial categories and used them to mark bodies as raced, thereby objectifying raced bodies via the creation of categories and then developing rational policies that involved the treatment of categories, not individuals.[25] This challenge to conceptions of modernity understands seemingly color-blind constructs as highly racialized—for example, claims that modernity itself as defined by the West is impossible without attending to race as a core feature of the definition and a new focus on the world system of the past five hundred years as a racialized one with implications for both the colonies and European nation-states.[26]

A final emphasis in critical race theory concerns its continued embrace of a social justice framework advanced by W. E. B. Du Bois and many others but now directed toward understanding and contesting the social inequalities that are obscured through color-blind racism. The visibility of color-coded systems of racial rule such as slavery, apartheid, and Jim Crow that created racial hierarchies were clear targets for scholars and activists committed to identifying the laws, norms, and institutions that perpetuated the system. The trajectory of critical race theory within legal studies illustrates this emphasis on addressing social inequalities as part of a broader social justice framework.[27] In the context of color-blind racism, the ideas and practices that create and reinforce racial hierarchies themselves become part of the apparatus of racism, which further complicates efforts to document and question social inequalities in racial terms.

Collectively, these analyses of color blindness have direct implications for analyzing the persisting centrality of race within bioscience. Because it conceals and rationalizes the social inequalities produced by institutional racism, color-blind racism presents new challenges for critical race theory. The thesis of race as socially constructed has been an important response in critical race theory to biologically based conceptions of race and provides a partial basis for examining scientific racism as a system of power. Within the social-constructionist framework, scientific institutions remain important to the creation and enforcement of racial ideologies. At the same time, the assumption that race as a biological construction has been discredited in the wake of the sustained attack on the premises of scientific racism may be overly optimistic.

As this book shows in the case of metabolic syndrome, racial difference is now being measured at the molecular level beneath the skin, a shift toward attaching racial meaning to biological objects in the body rather than on the surface of the skin.[28] Race remains a powerful tool to categorize human groups because it is now possible for scientists to author race using the languages of molecular and genetic difference.[29] The logic of color blindness takes multiple forms and involves scientists' use of a range of discursive strategies and scientific practices that aim to advance approaches to the study of human ancestry and susceptibility to disease that seem nonracial but that in fact are deeply racialized.

The discovery of DNA and the flourishing of molecular biology in the 1950s provided technological and discursive resources for scientists to shift away from using race and toward other ways of representing human difference. The cultural power of molecules such as DNA to define human difference became possible through molecularization (the ascendance of scientific institutions, procedures, and techniques that visualize, measure, and intervene in life at the molecular level) and through geneticization (the process through which differences between people are reduced to DNA codes).[30] As molecularization and geneticization sharpened the focus on DNA as a key prism for understanding human life, the hope was that race would no longer serve as a valid or useful biological classification for human beings. In 1990, the U.S. Department of Energy and the National Institutes of Health began what would later be named the Human Genome Project, a massive international research project whose primary goals were to identify the roughly thirty thousand genes and sequence the three billion base pairs that comprise human DNA. The field of population genetics was supposed to prove the scientific futility of race by demonstrating the overwhelming extent to which so-called races are genetically similar. Genetics had the cultural power to dislodge the false ideology of race by showing that more genetic variation exists *within* so-called racial groups than *between* racial groups.[31] In other words, racial categories did not map so neatly onto human DNA.

Science and technology (STS) scholars have emphasized that Western science gains cultural authority and manufactures scientific objectivity by concealing the institutional practices that construct scientific knowledges and the unequal power relationships in which those practices are embedded.[32] Through this process of concealment, molecularization provided scientists a process for conceptualizing human bodies in terms that were more consistent with the liberal priorities of Western biosciences. The scientific practices that comprise molecularization rose to prominence in a range of fields and signaled a new way of conceptualizing human differences that no longer explicitly required outward physical characteristics such as skin color. Thus, molecularization is consistent with broader efforts to promote a color-blind society.[33]

Catherine Bliss's ethnographic analysis of genomics experts suggests that while the field of genomics was initially organized around a color-blind approach to race during the period of its emergence from the post–World War II era to the mid-1990s, subsequent genomics researchers have worked to rearticulate genomics as a racially conscious and explicitly antiracist science.[34] Through bringing their own liberal antiracist politics to bear on the conduct of their science, genomics researchers sought to position genomics as the new scientific authority on race and a leading front in the struggle for social justice through a new ethical science.

In her examination of the resurgence of racial science, legal scholar Dorothy Roberts concludes that both liberal and conservative variations of color-blind racial politics draw on genomic meanings of race to advance their social policies. As she found in her interviews of genomic scientists, the liberal position is that race is biological and is a "neutral scientific fact that can be put to good or bad use and to advocate for safeguards against its misuse by racists."[35] For political conservatives, treating race as a proxy for genetic difference permits them to reject efforts to use political meanings of race to reform unjust social policies while simultaneously embracing bioscientific research that claims that blacks are genetically predisposed to crime. Roberts concludes that the redefinition of race as a genetic category naturalizes the social conditions created by contemporary racisms.

Other STS scholars have raised concerns by examining how race and biological truth are being reconfigured within the logic of color-blind racism. They continue to investigate ongoing forms of racially coded bioscience that combat the resurgence of scientific racism in several domains of inquiry—biomedical experimentation on African American prisoners, African Americans who take prescription drugs, for-profit companies that offer genetic ancestry tests that confirm existing racial categories, prescription drugs for treating heart disease, and teaching racial ideas about human biology.[36]

In the era of color blindness, racial essentialism still operates as a dominant epistemological framework for interpreting racial difference; however, it now can function without an explicit racial discourse. Instead, racial essentialism is transformed into highly technical discourses about population gene structure, risk, and familial genetic inheritance. This logic of color blindness defined the cultural power of the molecule and the gene to transform meanings of race in the new biosciences. Whereas prior forms of racial essentialism are routinely recognized as linked to color-consciousness, new dimensions of Western science associated with conditions of postmodernity are shaped by the logic of color blindness.

Scientists need to pay closer attention to new meanings of race within science and technology with an eye toward examining their potential implications for unjust power relations as defined by color-blind racism. It is unclear why it has been so difficult for contemporary race theories to incorporate these insights. One explanation for this conceptual blind spot is that the technical and discursive apparatuses that life scientists draw upon to construct new claims about the connections between race and biology have become quite elaborate. The disciplinary boundaries across the human and social sciences that foster niche specializations may obscure developments in other fields. The discourses of human genetics serve a gatekeeper function—the difficulties of entering into these expert discourses may represent a major impediment to contemporary race theorists.[37] While ideas from within critical race theory have been deployed to analyze the racial implications of federal science policies related to health, epidemiology and public health, and disparities in the medical treatment of racial and ethnic minorities, the exclusivity of these discourses might serve as one practical reason why racial justice advocates outside of the academy have been slow to challenge the resurgence of racial science.[38]

New forms of color-blind scientific racism, such as those represented by metabolic syndrome, are emerging in response to the color-conscious scientific racisms that defined modernity. Through their articulation in the logic of color blindness, these new forms of color-blind scientific racism serve to explain away the realities of extreme racially coded inequality. Racial inequalities and the globalized social structures that reproduce them are effaced by the logic of color blindness that has come to define postmodernity. If race served as an important conceptual anchor for the modern social order under conditions of postmodernity, color blindness now operates as a means of erasing that relationship by severing race discourses from the effects they produce. Repositioning race within the contemporary Western life sciences requires that race scholars rethink how the social practices of erasure might come to define the scientific racisms of the twenty-first century.

Critical race theory's partial neglect of science does not mean that science lacks race (or racism), but rather that critical analyses of science and technology have not been adequately integrated within critical race theory. However, there are also promising collaborations between bioscience and social science that are sensitive to the implications of genomics and molecularization for race and reflect a nuanced sociological understanding of how social categories such as race feed back into biological systems in complex ways.[39] Although bioscientists themselves are ultimately responsible for the racial meanings that inform and emerge from their scientific activities, critical race theorists also bear responsibility for penetrating bioscience with epistemological questions about how racial meanings are transformed. If race were no longer measured as a construct in bioscience research, it would be nearly impossible to document group-based inequalities that stem from institutional racism. Thus, race scholars must remain vigilant about the ongoing uses of race in bioscience and challenge racial sciences that affirm and justify racial subordination.

Prescriptions

I would like to conclude this book by offering a set of prescriptions for resistance and survival for groups of people struggling with metabolic health problems, and for those people who are currently positioned inside political and health institutions to act on our collective behalf. I am not a medical doctor, but as I have studied the science of metabolic syndrome and lived with diabetes myself for twenty-two years, I feel that I have useful information to offer people in similar circumstances. However, if social-science research produces valuable knowledge about right living, then I have a few prescriptions to offer that may prove useful. I understand that these recommendations may prove difficult for many people, especially those who work for a living—social class matters, too!

It is vital that people find ways to reject the industrialized food system in all its forms, especially mass-produced sugars and convenience foods.

We need to implement a kind of Birmingham bus boycott of all foods that requires laboratories, scientists, and factories for their mass production. This also includes all forms of fast food and much of what is available in America's chain grocery stores and restaurants. This boycott would target all foods that are produced under neoliberal food regimes that are exploiting farmers around the world, especially in former colonies, and creating global ecological disasters. We all deserve access to whole, organic foods, especially fruits, vegetables, and herbs. In addition to boycotting the industrialized food system, people should seek out and/or develop for themselves organic farmers' markets and community gardens where they live. Urban agriculture and sustainable food movements across the country are inspiring people to back sovereignty over the food system.

I began coming to consciousness about food politics in 2004 when I decided to stop eating fast food and try vegetarianism, in partial response to a doctor's visit that revealed moderately high LDL cholesterol levels and a politically astute and determined vegan friend. Immediately upon seeing the abnormal lab result, my endocrinologist wrote me a prescription for a cholesterol-lowering statin. After a brief confrontation prompted by my questions about whether or not we wanted to consider changes in my diet or exercise before a new medication (neither of which was ideal at the time), I left the prescription sitting on the examination table and decided to try something different. I am not suggesting that statins are wholly inappropriate or dangerous for others (these questions are beyond the scope of my expertise), but I was simply not ready to start taking a new drug without trying nondrug options first. In the intervening years, I have practiced vegetarianism, veganism, and paleo-inspired eating practices, and have not set foot inside a fast-food restaurant since.

We should become much better educated about the potential benefits and real dangers of all pharmaceuticals compared to nonpharmaceutical forms of healing and wellness. Prescription drugs represent a real and growing threat to Americans' health: overdoses and dosing errors are a leading cause of death in the United States and kill tens of thousands of people every year. While prescription drug therapy and other biomedical interventions are necessary in many instances, perhaps we, as a people, are turning to drugs too quickly to solve problems whose origins are not biological or biochemical, but social. In my view, the first step in *de*-medicalization is to look in our medicine cabinets and work with our doctors to rethink the absolute necessity of each drug on a case-by-case basis and consider viable alternatives to pharmacological solutions to metabolic problems. Yes, doctors are pillars of biomedicalization, and so it may seem counterintuitive to recommend that people work with them to extricate their bodies from the authority of those same medical officials. However, we have to start from a position that holds safety and wholeness as the primary features of a healing practice. If you happen to find yourself in a snake pit, leave *carefully*.

I cannot go back and tell the young brother on the MARC train what I know and what I've learned about surviving the politics of metabolism. I have come in contact with many people—family members, college students, strangers in the grocery store—who are suffering. I am suffering. I always experience a tinge of resentment when someone who knows I have diabetes says, "You can't eat that, can you?" I don't like the concept of policing food in the context of neoliberalism and its endless conversations about good choices. I turned in my own badge long ago; hence my silence on the train that morning.

We need to scrutinize and criticize the *systems of choices* for food and healing presented to us through the politics of metabolism. The convergence of technoscientific transformations within biomedicine, food systems, and pharmacopeia has created a context where people's bodies are the conduit for the extraction of scientific knowledge, agricultural surplus value, and drug company profits. We are the circuitry in the politics of metabolism, the nodes in a system of biopower that relies on our willingness to submit to routine biomedical testing, moral judgments about healthy choices, and mass consumption of unhealthy foods and unsafe medicines. We don't have to accept this arrangement as inevitable or permanent. I think our best chances for survival, for thriving within the politics of metabolism, lie in our commitments to teaching and helping each other heal outside these systems of government, corporation, and scientific institutions.

Like any book, this one was very much a cooperative endeavor. Without the human love, social support, and intellectual guidance of many people, *Blood Sugar* would not have been possible. I first offer thanksgiving to Rebekah, my dearest companion, who was the only high-school friend to visit me in the hospital when I was diagnosed with diabetes in 1992. Even then I knew our friendship was special, and indeed our time together on this earth continues to be a source of energy, purpose, and joy for me. I also thank my sweet children, Ruth and Elias, for sacrificing their playmate, short-order cook, and driver so that he could finish his book. I offer thanksgiving to Christine Hatch and Charles Hatch, my wonderful parents, for taking such good care of me, pointing me in the right direction in this country, and listening to my tirades and rambling about food over the years. Your selflessness never ceases to inspire me. I offer thanks for my sisters and brothers, Stephani Hatch Richards, Nicole Stargell, Willie Stargell Jr., and Marcus Richards, for being my loving shepherds and gently prodding me to walk my own path and speak my truth to the world. I offer thanksgiving for my family, both known and unknown, living and passed on. I directly thank M. F. L. T. and J. P. and all my brothers and sisters whose wisdom, power, and spirit resurrected the possibility of this project.

Quite literally, this book would not have been possible without the intellectual labor and personal commitment of my adviser and teacher Patricia Hill Collins. Her demands for excellence and clarity of thought transformed this project from a jumbled mess of ever-emerging ideas into something approximating sociology. I am forever grateful for her presence in my life at just the right time. At the University of Maryland, many other advisers helped shape this project in innumerable ways, especially Laura Mamo, Meyer Kestnbaum, George Ritzer, and Bonnie Thornton Dill. Meyer Kestnbaum's Work-in-Progress Seminar, of which I was a proud member, gave me the invaluable opportunity to develop my thinking in a rigorous public intellectual space. I offer special thanks for my homegirls at Maryland—Michelle Corbin, Emily Mann, and Kimberly Bonner—whose companionship, criticisms, and love continue to sustain me.

I offer thanks to the good people who make up and support the Minority Fellowship Program (MFP) at the American Sociological Association, especially Jean Shin, for honoring me by inviting me into the MFP family. The Minority Fellowship Program is a crowning jewel in American sociology, and I am truly grateful for the support this fellowship provided me as a doctoral student. Thanks to all of my former colleagues and students at Georgia State University for their support, with special thanks to Renee Shelby for her outstanding research assistance as I finished the manuscript. I thank my first sociology professor at Dartmouth College, Susan Thompson, who introduced me to the worlds of food security, social theory, and research methods, and to my friends and former colleagues at Emory University's Rollins School of Public Health for showing me how to integrate my passion for health education with the possibilities of social-science research. I also would like to thank Joyce Jacobsen and Joe Rouse at Wesleyan University and all of my new colleagues in the Science in Society Program for their belief in me and my work.

Finally, I offer thanksgiving to Jason Weidemann and the entire team at the University of Minnesota Press for seeing and believing in the promise of this project from day one. Thanks to Lundy Braun and to an anonymous reviewer for insightful and incisive comments that strengthened this book in ways I could not have envisioned. Any errors of fact or interpretation are my sole responsibility.

Preface

1. Glycated hemoglobin is also known as glycolated hemoglobin, glycosylated hemoglobin, hemoglobin A_{1c}, or HbA_{1c}.

2. These data were reported in the *Mortality and Morbidity Weekly Report* (MMWR) 56(43) (November 2, 2007): 1133–37. The racial categories in the BRFSS are statutorily based on the Office of Management and Budget's (OMB's) 1997 "Standards for Maintaining, Collecting, and Presenting Federal Data on Race and Ethnicity," *Federal Register* 62 (1997): 58781–90. The OMB recommendations on the measurement of race and ethnicity in the general population note that "the [racial] categories that were developed represent a social-political construct designed to be used in the collection of data on the race and ethnicity of major broad population groups in this country, and are not anthropologically or scientifically based" (36874).

3. Elevated blood pressure, or hypertension, is defined as systolic pressure of at least 140 mmHg and diastolic pressure of at least 90 mmHg. Elevated cholesterol, or dyslipidemia, is defined as total serum cholesterol higher than 240. Elevated blood sugar, or hyperglycemia, is defined as fasting blood glucose of at least 126 mg/dL. Elevated weight, or obesity, is defined as a body mass index (BMI) greater than 30.

Introduction

1. http://www.nlm.nih.gov/medlineplus/ency/article/002257.htm (accessed August 22, 2006).

2. Bernard C. K. Choi, David J. Hunter, Walter Tsou, and Peter Sainsbury, "Diseases of Comfort: Primary Cause of Death in the 22nd Century," *Journal of Epidemiology and Community Health* 59 (2005): 1030–34.

3. Majid Ezzati, Stephen Vander Hoorn, Carlene M. M. Lawes, Rachel Leach, W. Philip T. James, Alan D. Lopez, Anthony Rodgers, and Christopher J. L. Murray, "Rethinking the 'Diseases of Affluence' Paradigm: Global Patterns of Nutritional Risks in Relation to Economic Development," *PLoS Medicine* 2 (2005): e133.

4. S. Jay Olshansky and A. Brian Ault, "The Fourth Stage of the Epidemiologic Transition: The Age of Delayed Degenerative Diseases," *Milbank Quarterly* 64 (1986): 355–91; Abdel R. Omran, "The Epidemiologic Transition: A Theory of the Epidemiology of Population Change," *Milbank Quarterly* 83 (2005): 731–57; Abdel R. Omran, "The Epidemiologic Transition: A Theory of the Epidemiology of Population Change," *Milbank Memorial Fund Quarterly* 49 (1971): 509–38.

5. For introductory purposes, I use the term "metabolic syndrome" as an umbrella term to encompass many different concepts advanced by biomedical researchers to describe these relations, including metabolic syndrome, dysmetabolic syndrome X, insulin resistance syndrome, and syndrome X.

6. Elevated blood pressure, or hypertension, is defined as having systolic pressure of at least 140 mmHg and diastolic pressure of at least 90 mmHg. Elevated cholesterol, or dyslipidemia, is defined as having total serum cholesterol higher than 240. Elevated blood sugar, or hyperglycemia, is defined as having fasting blood glucose of at least 126 mg/dL. Elevated weight, or obesity, is defined as having a body mass index (BMI) greater than 30.

7. W. Dallas Hall, Jackson T. Wright, Ella W. Horton, Shiriki K. Kumanyika, Luther T. Clark, Nanette K. Wenger, Keith C. Ferdinand, Karol Watson, and John M. Flack, "The Metabolic Syndrome in African Americans: A Review," *Ethnicity and Disease* 13 (2003): 414–28.

8. Earl S. Ford, Wayne H. Giles, and William H. Dietz, "Prevalence of the Metabolic Syndrome among US Adults: Findings from the Third National Health and Nutrition Examination Survey," *Journal of the American Medical Association* 287 (2002): 356–59. The definition of metabolic syndrome used in this analysis was from the National Cholesterol Education Program (NCEP), which will be discussed along with the NHANES study in chapter 2. I conducted a works-cited search for the Ford et al. study on December 11, 2006, in the Expanded Science Citations Index (ISI Web of Science) and found 1,114 articles published between 2002 and 2006 that cited this study. By August 20, 2008, 1,676 articles cited this article, increasing by 562 citations in less than two years.

9. http://www.metabolicsyndromeinstitute.com/about/mission (accessed March 5, 2009).

10. Gerald Reaven, Terry Kristen Strom, and Barry Fox, *Syndrome X: The Silent Killer: The New Heart Disease Risk* (New York: Simon & Schuster, 2000); Scott M. Grundy, *Contemporary Diagnosis and Management of the Metabolic Syndrome* (Newton, Pa.: Handbooks in Health Care, 2005); Scott D. Mendelson, *Metabolic Syndrome and Psychiatric Illness: Interaction, Pathophysiology, Assess-*

ment, and Treatment (San Diego: Academic Press, 2008); Barbara Caleen Hansen and George A. Bray, *The Metabolic Syndrome: Epidemiology, Clinical Treatment, and Underlying Mechanisms* (Totowa, N.J.: Humana Press 2008).

11. This is based on a search I conducted of the ISI Web of Science bibliographic database on February 5, 2007, and again on October 15, 2008, for the terms "metabolic syndrome," "insulin resistance syndrome," "syndrome X," and "dys-metabolic syndrome X." This search showed that 16,040 original research articles were published on the metabolic syndrome and related terms between 1962 and 2007.

12. For more on the proposed relationships between components of the meta-bolic syndrome and kidney and liver disease, see E. Bugianesi, A. J. McCullough, and G. Marchesini, "Insulin Resistance: A Metabolic Pathway to Chronic Liver Disease," *Hepatology* 42 (2005): 987–1000; J. Chen, P. Muntner, L. L. Hamm, D. W. Jones, V. Batuman, V. Fonseca, P. K. Whelton, and J. He, "The Metabolic Syndrome and Chronic Kidney Disease in US Adults," *Annals of Internal Medicine* 140 (2004): 167–74; M. Kurella, J. C. Lo, and G. M. Chertow, "Metabolic Syndrome and the Risk for Chronic Kidney Disease among Nondiabetic Adults," *Journal of the American Society of Nephrology* 16 (2005): 2134–40; and P. Muntner, J. He, J. Chen, V. Fonseca, and P. K. Whelton, "Prevalence of Non-traditional Cardio-vascular Disease Risks Factors among Persons with Impaired Fasting Glucose, Impaired Glucose Tolerance, Diabetes, and the Metabolic Syndrome: Analysis of the Third Health and Nutrition Examination Survey (NHANES III)," *Annals of Epidemiology* 14 (2004): 686–95. For more on the proposed relationship be-tween components of metabolic syndrome and polycystic ovarian syndrome, see D. Apter, T. Butzow, G. A. Laughlin, and S. S. C. Yen, "Metabolic Features of Polycystic-Ovary-Syndrome Are Found in Adolescent Girls with Hyperandrogen-ism," *Journal of Clinical Endocrinology and Metabolism* 80 (1995): 2966–73; C. J. Glueck, J. R. Papanna, P. Wang, N. Goldenberg, and L. Sieve-Smith, "Inci-dence and Treatment of Metabolic Syndrome in Newly Referred Women with Confirmed Polycystic Ovarian Syndrome," *Metabolism-Clinical and Experimen-tal* 52 (2003): 908–15; A. J. Morales, G. A. Laughlin, T. Butzow, H. Maheshwari, G. Baumann, and S. S. C. Yen, "Insulin, Somatotropic, and Luteinizing Hormone Axes in Lean and Obese Women with Polycystic Ovary Syndrome: Common and Distinct Features," *Journal of Clinical Endocrinology and Metabolism* 81 (1996): 2854–64; and C. G. Solomon, "The Epidemiology of Polycystic Ovary Syndrome—Prevalence and Associated Disease Risk," *Endocrinology and Metabolism Clinics of North America* 28 (1999): 247. For more on the proposed relationships be-tween components of metabolic syndrome and breast and colorectal cancer, see J. M. Argiles and F. J. Lopez-Soriano, "Insulin and Cancer," *International Journal of Oncology* 18 (2001): 683–87; P. F. Bruning, J. M. G. Bonfret, P. A. H. Van Nooyrd, A. A Hart, M. De Jong-Bakker, and W. J. Noojen, "Insulin Resistance and

Breast Cancer Risk," *International Journal of Cancer* 52 (1992): 511–16; C. La Vecchia, E. Negri, A. Decarli, and S. Frabceschi, "Diabetes Mellitus and Colorectal Cancer Risk," *Cancer Epidemiology and Biomarkers Prevention* 6 (1997): 1007–10; and J. C. Will, D. A. Galuska, F. Vinicor, and E E. Calle, "Colorectal Cancer: Another Complication of Diabetes Mellitus?" *American Journal of Epidemiology* 147 (1998): 816–25. For more on the proposed relationship between components of metabolic syndrome and HIV infection, see C. Hadigan, J. B. Meigs, C. Corcoran, P. Rietschel, S. Piecuch, N. Basgoz, B. Davis, P. Sax, T. Stanley, P. W. F. Wilson, R. B. D'Agostino, and S. Grinspoon, "Metabolic Abnormalities and Cardiovascular Disease Risk Factors in Adults with Human ImmunoDeficiency Virus Infection and Lipodystrophy," *Clinical Infectious Diseases* 32 (2001): 130–39; H. Murata, P. W. Hruz, and M. Mueckler, "The Mechanism of Insulin Resistance Caused by HIV Protease Inhibitor Therapy," *Journal of Biological Chemistry* 275 (2000): 20251–54; and S. Safrin and C. Grunfeld, "Fat Distribution and Metabolic Changes in Patients with HIV Infection," *Aids* 13 (1999): 2493–2505. For more on the proposed relationships between components of metabolic syndrome and erectile dysfunction, see T. C. Bansal, A. T. Guay, J. Jacobson, B. O. Woods, and R. W. Nesto, "Incidence of Metabolic Syndrome and Insulin Resistance in a Population with Organic Erectile Dysfunction," *Journal of Sexual Medicine* 2 (2005): 96–103; A. Guay, and J. Jacobson, "The Relationship between Testosterone Levels, the Metabolic Syndrome (by Two Criteria), and Insulin Resistance in a Population of Men with Organic Erectile Dysfunction," *Journal of Sexual Medicine* 4 (2007): 1046–55; S. A. Kaplan, A. G. Meehan, and A. Shah, "The Age Related Decrease in Testosterone Is Significantly Exacerbated in Obese Men with the Metabolic Syndrome. What Are the Implications for the Relatively High Incidence of Erectile Dysfunction Observed in These Men?" *Journal of Urology* 176 (2006): 1524–27; V. Kupelian, R. Shabsigh, A. B. Araujo, A. B. O'Donnell, and J. B. McKinlay, "Erectile Dysfunction as a Predictor of the Metabolic Syndrome in Aging Men: Results from the Massachusetts Male Aging Study," *Journal of Urology* 176 (2006): 222–26; and N. Makhsida, J. Shah, G. Yan, H. Fisch, and R. Shabsigh, "Hypogonadism and Metabolic Syndrome: Implications for Testosterone Therapy," *Journal of Urology* 174 (2005): 827–34.

13. A more extensive discussion of this topic can be found in chapter 2.

14. A more extensive discussion of this topic can be found in chapter 4. For more on the proposed relationships between the components of the metabolic syndrome and mental illness, see my analysis of schizophrenia and antipsychotics in chapter 4 and see also R. A. Bermudes, P. E. Keck, and J. A. Welge, "The Prevalence of the Metabolic Syndrome in Psychiatric Inpatients with Primary Psychotic and Mood Disorders," *Psychosomatics* 47 (2006): 491–97; T. Heiskanen, L. Niskanen, R. Lyytikainen, P. I. Saarinen, and J. Hintikka, "Metabolic Syndrome in Patients with Schizophrenia," *Journal of Clinical Psychiatry* 64 (2003): 575–79; Harvard Mental Health, "Schizophrenia and the Metabolic Syndrome," *Harvard*

Mental Health Letter 23 (October 2006); Gary Remington, "Schizophrenia, Antipsychotics, and the Metabolic Syndrome: Is There a Silver Lining?" *American Journal of Psychiatry* 163 (2006): 1132–34; and Jogin H. Thakore, "Metabolic Syndrome and Schizophrenia," *British Journal of Psychiatry* 186 (2005): 455–56.

15. I analyze the NCEP's definition of the metabolic syndrome in greater detail in chapter 2.

16. This search included the terms "metabolic syndrome," "dysmetabolic syndrome X," "syndrome X," and "insulin resistance syndrome." The search was conducted on October 24, 2013.

17. This data was accessed on IMS Health.com, a global leader in pharmaceutical industry information, on April 5, 2009: http://www.imshealth.com/portal/site/imshealth/menuitem.a46c6d4df3db4b3d88f611019418c22a/?vgnextoid=841365272046e110VgnVCM100000ed152ca2RCRD.

18. http://static.correofarmaceutico.com/docs/2013/05/20/usareport.pdf (accessed October 20, 2013). IMS Institute for Healthcare Informatics, "Declining Medicine Use and Costs: For Better or Worse" (Parsippany, N.J.: IMS Institute for Healthcare Informatics, May 2015).

19. http://www.firstwordpharma.com/node/1096220#axzz2iN3I9KHx (accessed October 21, 2013). The other metabolic drugs were #2 Plavix (9.92 billion), #9 Crestor (6.62 billion), #10 Lantus (6.38 billion), #14 Diovan (6.05 billion), and #17 Zocor (5.5445 billion).

20. Michel Foucault defined the apparatus as the heterogeneous network of power and knowledge that can be established between discourses (including scientific, philosophic, moral, and philanthropic statements), institutions, structural arrangements, policy decisions, laws, and administrative measures. See Michel Foucault, *The Essential Foucault,* ed. P. Rabinow and N. Rose (New York: New Press, 2003).

21. Scott M. Grundy, "Metabolic Syndrome Pandemic," *Arteriosclerosis Thrombosis and Vascular Biology* 28 (2008): 629–36; Dean J. Kereiakes and James T. Willerson, "Metabolic Syndrome Epidemic," *Circulation* 108 (2003): 1552–53; P. Zimmet, K. G. Alberti, and J. Shaw, "Global and Societal Implications of the Diabetes Epidemic," *Nature* 414 (2001): 782–87.

22. Michel Foucault, *Society Must Be Defended: Lectures at the Collège de France, 1975–1976,* ed. François Ewald, Alessandro Fontana, and Mauro Bertani, trans. David Macey (New York: Picador, 2003 [1976]), 244.

23. Direct costs include the costs of physicians and other professionals, hospital and nursing-home services, the cost of medications, home health care, and other medical goods. Indirect costs refer to lost economic productivity because of premature disease and death. This estimate is compiled from the following sources: American Diabetes Association, "Economic Costs of Diabetes in the U.S. in 2002," *Diabetes Care* 26 (2002): 917–32; Eric A. Finkelstein, Christopher J. Ruhm, and Katherine M. Kosa, "Economic Causes and Consequences of Obesity,"

Annual Review of Public Health 26 (2005): 239–57; and Thomas Thom, "Heart Disease and Stroke Statistics—2006 Update: A Report from the American Heart Association Statistics Committee and Stroke Statistics Subcommittee," *Circulation* 113 (2006): e85–e151.

24. In 1997, the Office of Management and Budget (OMB) provided the definitions of race and ethnicity that must be used in all biomedical and health-policy research funded by the federal government. See Steve Epstein, *Inclusion: The Politics of Difference in Medical Research* (Chicago: University of Chicago Press, 2007); and Alexandra E. Shields, Michael Fortun, Evelyn M. Hammonds, Patricia A. King, Caryn Lerman, Rayna Rapp, and Patrick F. Sullivan, "The Use of Race Variables in Genetic Studies of Complex Traits and the Goal of Reducing Health Disparities," *American Psychologist* 60 (2005): 77–103.

25. For analyses of this research, see chapter 3.

26. Office of Management and Budget, "Standards for Maintaining, Collecting, and Presenting Federal Data on Race and Ethnicity," *Federal Register* 62 (1997): 58781–90.

27. Ibid., 36874.

28. See David S. Jones and Roy H. Perlis, "Pharmacogenetics, Race, and Psychiatry: Prospects and Challenges," *Harvard Review of Psychiatry* 14 (2006): 92; Jonathan T. Kahn, "Race, Pharmacogenomics and Marketing Putting BiDil in Context," *American Journal of Bioethics* 6 (2006): W1–W5; and Sandra Soo-Jin Lee, "Racializing Drug Design: Implications of Pharmacogenomics for Health Disparities," *American Journal of Public Health* 95 (2005): 2133–38.

29. J. M. Flack, R. Victor, K. Watson, K. C. Ferdinand, E. Saunders, L. Tarasenko, M. J. Jamieson, H. Shi, and P. Bruschi, "Improved Attainment of Blood Pressure and Cholesterol Goals Using Single-Pill Amlodipine/Atorvastatin in African Americans: The CAPABLE Trial," *Mayo Clinic Proceedings* 83 (2008): 35–45.

30. Ibid.

31. Troy Duster, "Race and Reification in Science," *Science* 307 (2005): 1050–51; Jonathan T. Kahn, "Race, Pharmacogenomics and Marketing Putting BiDil in Context," *American Journal of Bioethics* 6 (2006): W1–W5; Jonathan Kahn, *Race in a Bottle: The Story of BiDil and Racialized Medicine in a Post-Genomic Age* (New York: Columbia University Press, 2012); and Pamela Sankar and Jonathan Kahn, "BiDil: Race Medicine or Race Marketing?" *Health Affairs* (2005): 54–55.

32. See my analysis in chapter 4.

33. Centers for Disease Control and Prevention, "Racial/Ethnic and Socioeconomic Disparities in Multiple Risk Factors for Heart Disease and Stroke—United States, 2003," *Mortality and Morbidity Weekly Report* 54 (2005): 113–17.

34. David R. Williams and Michelle Sternthal, "Understanding Racial-Ethnic Disparities in Health: Sociological Contributions," *Journal of Health and Social Behavior* 51 (2010): S15–S27.

35. I. J. Benjamin, D. K. Arnett, and J. Loscalzo, "Discovering the Full Spectrum

of Cardiovascular Disease Minority Health Summit 2003—Report of the Basic Science Writing Group," *Circulation* 111 (2005): E120–E123; A. H. Mokdad, J. S. Marks, D. F. Stroup, and J. L. Gerberding, "Actual Causes of Death in the United States, 2000," *Journal of the American Medical Association* 291 (2004): 1238–45; Qi Zhang and Youfa Wang, "Trends in the Association between Obesity and Socioeconomic Status in U.S. Adults: 1971 to 2000," *Obesity Research* 12 (2004): 1622–32; Raynard S. Kington, and James P. Smith, "Socioeconomic Status and Racial and Ethnic Differences in Functional Status Associated with Chronic Diseases," *American Journal of Public Health* 87 (1997): 805–10; Michael G. Marmot, "Understanding Social Inequalities in Health," *Perspectives in Biology and Medicine* 46 (2003): S9–S23; Mark D. Hayward, Eileen M. Crimmins, Toni P. Miles, and Yu Yang, "The Significance of Socioeconomic Status in Explaining the Race Gap in Chronic Health Conditions," *American Sociological Review* 65(6) (2000): 910–30; J. C. Phelan and B. G. Link, "Controlling Disease and Creating Disparities: A Fundamental Cause Perspective," *Journal of Gerontology* 60B (2005): 27–33.

36. Michel Foucault, *The History of Sexuality: An Introduction: Volume I,* trans. Robert Hurley (New York: Vintage Books, 1978), 101–2.

37. In terms of Foucault's own scholarship, there are a few key sources for Foucault's ideas about genealogical historiography: Michel Foucault, *The Archaeology of Knowledge and the Discourse on Language,* trans. Alan M. Sheridan Smith (New York: Pantheon Books, 1972); Foucault, *The History of Sexuality*; Michel Foucault, *Power/Knowledge: Selected Interviews and Other Writings, 1972–1977,* ed. C. Gordon, trans. C. Gordon, L. Marshall, J. Mepham, and K. Soper (New York: Pantheon Books, 1980); and Foucault, *The Essential Foucault.* There are too many secondary interpretations of the genealogical method to mention here, but I relied especially on the following: Arnold I. Davidson, "Archaeology, Genealogy, Ethics," in *Foucault: A Critical Reader,* ed. D. C. Hoy (Oxford: Basil Blackwell, 1986), 221–34; Michael Mahon, *Foucault's Nietzschean Genealogy: Truth, Power, and the Subject* (Albany: State University of New York Press, 1992); Rudi Visker, *Michel Foucault: Genealogy as Critique,* trans. C. Turner (London: Verso, 1995); Mitchell Dean, *Critical and Effective Histories: Foucault's Methods and Historical Sociology* (London: Routledge, 1994); H. L. Drefus and Paul Rabinow, *Michel Foucault: Beyond Structuralism and Hermeneutics* (New York: Harvester Wheatsheaf, 1982); Todd May, *Between Genealogy and Epistemology: Psychology, Politics, and Knowledge in the Thought of Michel Foucault* (Philadelphia: Pennsylvania State University Press, 1993).

38. Scholars and theorists from a range of disciplines have attempted to craft a clear conception of what genealogy entails. For this discussion, see Dean, *Critical and Effective Histories*; Gavin Kendall and Gary Wickham, *Using Foucault's Methods* (Thousand Oaks, Calif.: Sage Publications, 1999); Scott Lash, "Genealogy and the Body: Foucault/Deleuze/Nietzsche," *Theory, Culture, and Society* 2

(1984): 1–17; Neil Levy, "History as Struggle: Foucault's Genealogy of Genealogy," *History of the Human Sciences* 11 (1998): 159–70; Michael Mahon, *Foucault's Nietzschean Genealogy: Truth, Power, and the Subject* (Albany: State University of New York Press, 1992); May, *Between Genealogy and Epistemology*; Daphne Meadmore, Caroline Hatcher, and Eric McWilliam, "Getting Tense about Genealogy," *Qualitative Studies in Education* 13 (2000): 463–76; C. G. Prado, *Starting with Foucault: An Introduction to Genealogy* (Boulder, Colo.: Westview Press, 2000); Ben Sax, "On the Genealogical Method: Nietzsche and Foucault," *International Studies in Philosophy* 22 (1990): 129–41; Larry Shiner, "Reading Foucault: Anti-Method and the Genealogy of Power-Knowledge," *History and Theory* 21 (1982): 382–98; and Visker, *Michel Foucault*.

39. Michel Foucault, "Nietzsche, Genealogy, History," in *The Essential Foucault,* 351–69; Foucault, *Society Must Be Defended*; May, *Between Genealogy and Epistemology*.

40. Michel Foucault, "Questions of Method," in *The Essential Foucault,* 248.

41. Dean, *Critical and Effective Histories,* 28.

42. Foucault euphemistically calls this network of power/knowledge relationships the "hazardous play of dominations" (Foucault, "Nietzsche, Genealogy, History," 357). In his thinking, this play of dominations manifests itself in the rituals and practices of bodies and laws and regulations that impose various rights and obligations on bodies (351–69).

43. Michel Foucault, *The Birth of the Clinic: An Archaeology of Medical Perception,* trans. Alan M. Sheridan Smith (New York: Vintage Books, 1975).

44. Foucault, *Society Must Be Defended,* 30.

45. Adele E. Clarke, *Situational Analysis: Grounded Theory after the Postmodern Turn* (Thousand Oaks, Calif.: Sage Publications, 2005).

46. Karl Marx, *Capital: A New Abridgment,* ed. David McLellan (Oxford: Oxford University Press, 1995), 43–44.

47. Donna J. Haraway, *Modest_Witness@Second_Millennium.FemaleMan_Meets_Oncomouse* (New York: Routledge, 1997), 135.

48. Michel Foucault defines a discursive formation as a series of regularities or patterns in statements in terms of the objects to which they refer, the concepts used, and the thematic choices that circumscribe them over time. See Foucault, *The Archaeology of Knowledge and the Discourse on Language,* 38.

1. Race, Biomedicine, and Health Injustice

1. Patricia Collins, *Fighting Words: Black Women and the Search for Justice* (Minneapolis: University of Minnesota Press, 1998).

2. Michael Omi and Howard Winant, *Racial Formation in the United States* (New York: Routledge, 1994), 55.

3. Anne McClintock, *Imperial Leather: Race, Gender, and Sexuality in the Colonial Contest* (New York: Routledge, 1995); Laura Ann Stoler, *Race and the Education of Desire: Foucault's History of Sexuality and the Colonial Order of Things* (Durham, N.C.: Duke University Press, 1995); David Theo Goldberg, *The Racial State* (Malden, Mass.: Blackwell Publishers, 2002); Howard Winant, *The World Is a Ghetto: Race and Democracy since World War II* (New York: Basic Books, 2001); Elazar Barkan, *The Retreat of Scientific Racism: Changing Concepts of Race in Britain and the United States between the World Wars* (New York: Cambridge University Press, 1992); Troy Duster, "Buried Alive: The Concept of Race in Science," in *Genetic Nature/Culture: Anthropology and Science beyond the Two-Culture Divide,* ed. A. H. Goodman, D. Heath, and M. S. Lindee (Berkeley and London: University of California Press, 2003), 258–77; Joseph L. Graves Jr., *The Emperor's New Clothes: Biological Theories of Race at the Millennium* (New Brunswick, N.J.: Rutgers University Press, 2001); Nancy Leys Stepan, *The Idea of Race in Science: Great Britain 1800–1960* (Hamden, Conn.: Archon Books, 1982).

4. Eduardo Bonilla-Silva, "Rethinking Racism: Toward a Structural Interpretation," *American Sociological Review* 62 (1997): 465–80; Stokely Carmichael and Charles V. Hamilton, *Black Power: The Politics of Liberation in America* (New York: Vintage Books, 1967).

5. Michael K. Brown, Martin Carnoy, Elliott Currie, Troy Duster, David B. Oppennheimer, Majorie M. Shultz, and David Wellman, *Whitewashing Race: The Myth of a Color-Blind Society* (Berkeley: University of California Press, 2003).

6. Ibid.; Lani Guinier and Gerald Torres, *The Miner's Canary: Enlisting Race, Resisting Power, Transforming Democracy* (Cambridge: Harvard University Press, 2002); Thomas M. Shapiro, *The Hidden Costs of Being African American: How Wealth Perpetuates Inequality* (New York: Oxford University Press, 2004); Evelyn Nakano Glenn, *Unequal Freedom: How Race and Gender Shaped American Citizenship and Labor* (Cambridge: Harvard University Press, 2002); Michelle Alexander, *The New Jim Crow: Mass Incarceration in the Age of Jim Crow* (New York: New Press, 2010).

7. Omi and Winant, *Racial Formation in the United States.*

8. Ibid., 57.

9. Ibid., 56.

10. Winant, *The World Is a Ghetto.*

11. Anthony R. Hatch, "Transformations of Race in Science: Critical Race Theory, Scientific Racism, and the Logic of Colorblindness," *Issues in Race and Society* 2 (2014): 7–41.

12. There is a voluminous body of knowledge about the history, philosophy, and politics of race in science over the past two decades. Some outstanding sources on these issues are Troy Duster, *Backdoor to Eugenics,* 2d ed. (New York:

Routledge, 2003 [1990]); Graves, *The Emperor's New Clothes*; Sandra Harding, *The "Racial" Economy of Science: Toward a Democratic Future* (Bloomington: Indiana University Press, 1993); Diane B. Paul, *The Politics of Heredity: Essays on Eugenics, Biomedicine, and the Nature–Nurture Debate* (Albany: State University of New York Press, 1998); Stepan, *The Idea of Race in Science*; and Naomi Zack, *Philosophy of Science and Race* (London: Routledge, 2002).

13. Harriet A. Washington, *Medical Apartheid: The Dark History of Medical Experimentation on Black Americans from Colonial Times to the Present* (New York: Doubleday, 2006).

14. On science and institutional racial power, see Paolo Palladino and Michael Worboys, "Science and Imperialism," *Isis* 84(1) (1993): 91–102; Craig Steven Wilder, *Ebony and Ivy: Race, Slavery, and the Troubled History of America's Universities* (New York: Bloomsbury, 2013). On racial fictions in science, see Ashley Montagu, *Man's Most Dangerous Myth: The Fallacy of Race*, 5th ed. (London: Oxford University Press, 1974); Audrey Smedley and Brian Smedley, "Race as Biology Is Fiction, Racism as Social Problem Is Real," *American Psychologist* 60(1) (2005): 16–26.

15. Daniel Kevles, *In the Name of Eugenics: Genetics and the Uses of Human Heredity* (Berkeley: University of California Press, 1985); Paul, *The Politics of Heredity*; Tukufu Zuberi, *Thicker Than Blood: An Essay on How Racial Statistics Lie* (Minneapolis: University of Minnesota Press, 2001).

16. This is the shift that historian Elazar Barkan famously described as the retreat of scientific racism, which refers to physical anthropology's adoption of the concepts, methods, and theories of population genetics (Barkan, *The Retreat of Scientific Racism*).

17. Jennifer Reardon, *Race to the Finish: Identity and Governance in an Age of Genomics* (Princeton, N.J.: Princeton University Press, 2005).

18. Institute of Medicine, *Unequal Treatment: Understanding Racial and Ethnic Disparities in Health* (Washington, D.C.: Institute of Medicine, 2002).

19. Reardon, *Race to the Finish*.

20. Ibid.

21. United Nations Educational, Scientific and Cultural Organization, *The Race Question*, vol. 3 (Paris: United Nations Educational, Scientific and Cultural Organization, 1950), 6.

22. Winant, *The World Is a Ghetto*, 296.

23. In a more lyrical way, Goldberg explains that "the 'primitive' is the romantic fabrication of and longing for an original human subjectivity, pristine in its representation" (*The Racial State*, 202). For more on scientific discourses of primitivism, see Donna J. Haraway, *Primate Visions: Gender, Race, and Nature in the World of Modern Science* (New York: Routledge, 1989).

24. At least since Omi and Winant, contemporary critical race theorists have

recognized the centrality of the state to racial formation. See Goldberg, *The Racial State*; Omi and Winant, *Racial Formation in the United States*; and Jacqueline Stevens, "Racial Meanings and Scientific Methods: Changing Policies for NIH-Sponsored Publications Reporting Human Variation," *Journal of Health Politics, Policy and Law* 28 (2003): 1033–87.

25. The 1790 census asked five questions: the number of free white males over sixteen years old, free white males under sixteen, free white females, other, and number of slaves.

26. Office of Management and Budget, "Standards for Maintaining, Collecting, and Presenting Federal Data on Race and Ethnicity," *Federal Register* 62 (1997): 58781–90.

27. Steven Epstein, *Inclusion: The Politics of Difference in Medical Research* (Chicago: University of Chicago Press, 2007); Stevens, "Racial Meanings and Scientific Methods," 1033–87.

28. National Institutes of Health, "NIH Guidelines for Inclusion of Women and Minorities as Subjects in Clinical Research" (2001), http:grants.nih.gov/grants/funding/women_min/guidelines_amended_10_2001.htm (accessed February 1, 2007). The Food and Drug Administration enforces similar guidelines regarding the inclusion of women and racial minorities in drug clinical trials.

29. Adele E. Clarke, Laura Mamo, Jennifer R. Fishman, Janet K. Shim, and Jennifer Ruth Fosket, "Biomedicalization: Technoscientific Transformations of Health, Illness, and U.S. Biomedicine," *American Sociological Review* 68 (2003): 161–94.

30. Paul Starr, *The Social Transformation of American Medicine: The Rise of a Sovereign Profession and the Making of a Vast Industry* (New York: Basic Books, 1982); Peter Conrad, *The Medicalization of Society* (Baltimore: Johns Hopkins University Press, 2007).

31. Donna J. Haraway, *Modest_Witness@Second_Millennium.FemaleMan_Meets_OncoMouse* (New York: Routledge, 1997); Bruno Latour, *Science in Action: How to Follow Scientists and Engineers through Society* (Cambridge: Harvard University Press, 1987).

32. Haraway, *Modest_Witness@Second_Millennium.FemaleMan_Meets_Onco Mouse*; Sheila Jasanoff, *States of Knowledge: The Co-production of Science and the Social Order* (London: Routledge, 2004); Nelly Oudshoorn, *Beyond the Natural Body: An Archeology of Sex Hormones* (London: Routledge, 2002).

33. Oudshoorn, *Beyond the Natural Body*, 13.

34. Lily Kay, *The Molecular Vision of Life: Caltech, the Rockefeller Foundation, and the New Biology* (New York: Oxford University Press, 1993); Nikolas Rose, "The Politics of Life Itself," *Theory, Culture, and Society* 18 (2001): 1–13; Sara Shostak, "Environmental Justice and Genomics: Acting on the Futures of Environmental Health," *Science as Culture* 13 (2004): 539–62.

35. Abby Lippman, "Prenatal Genetic Testing and Screening: Constructing Needs and Reinforcing Inequities," *American Journal of Law and Medicine* 17 (1991): 15–50.

36. Shostak, "Environmental Justice and Genomics," 539–62.

37. Ibid., 547.

38. Mervyn Susser, "Does Risk Factor Epidemiology Put Epidemiology at Risk? Peering into the Future," *Journal of Epidemiology and Community Health* 63 (1998): 608–11; Mervyn Susser and Ezra Susser, "Choosing a Future for Epidemiology: I. Eras and Paradigms," *American Journal of Public Health* 86 (1996): 668–73; Mervyn Susser and Ezra Susser, "Choosing a Future for Epidemiology: II. From Black Box to Chinese Boxes and Eco-Epidemiology," *American Journal of Public Health* 86 (1996): 674–77.

39. Clarke, Mamo, Fishman, Shim, and Fosket, "Biomedicalization," 161–94.

40. Adam Hegecoe, *The Politics of Personalized Medicine: Pharmacogenetics in the Clinic* (Cambridge: Cambridge University Press, 2004); Michael Kremer and Rachel Glennerster, *Strong Medicine: Creating Incentives for Pharmaceutical Research on Neglected Diseases* (Princeton, N.J.: Princeton University Press, 2004); Ray Moynihan, Iona Heath, and David Henry, "Selling Sickness: The Pharmaceutical Industry and Disease Mongering," *British Medical Journal* 324 (2002): 886–91.

41. Nikolas Rose, *The Politics of Life Itself* (Princeton, N.J.: Princeton University Press, 2006); Robert Mitchell and Catherine Waldby, "National Biobanks: Clinical Labor, Risk Production, and the Creation of Biovalue," *Science, Technology, and Human Values* 35:3 (2010): 330–55.

42. Charis Thompson, *Making Parents: The Ontological Choreography of Reproductive Technologies* (Cambridge: MIT Press, 2006).

43. Henry Etzkowitz, Peter Healey, and Andrew Webster, *Capitalizing Knowledge: New Intersections of Industry and Academia* (Albany: State University of New York Press, 1998); John P. Swann, *Academic Scientists and the Pharmaceutical Industry: Cooperative Research in Twentieth-Century America* (Baltimore: Johns Hopkins University Press, 1988); G. Teeling-Smith, *Science, Industry, and the State* (Oxford: Pergamon Press, 1965).

44. Sandra Soo-Jin Lee, "Racializing Drug Design: Implications of Pharmacogenomics for Health Disparities," *American Journal of Public Health* 95 (2005): 2133–38. Several other scholars have examined the use of race and ethnicity in pharmacological research and development. See Troy Duster, "Race and Reification in Science," *Science* 307 (2005): 1050–51; Lisa Gannett, "Group Categories in Pharmacogenetics Research," *Philosophy of Science* 72 (2005): 1232–47; and Pamela Sankar and Jonathan Kahn, "BiDil: Race Medicine or Race Marketing?" *Health Affairs* (October 11, 2005): 54–55.

45. Michel Foucault, *The History of Sexuality: An Introduction: Volume I,* trans. Robert Hurley (New York: Vintage Books, 1978), 140.

46. Michel Foucault, *Discipline and Punish: The Birth of the Prison,* trans. Alan M. Sheridan Smith (New York: Vintage Books, 1975).

47. Todd May, *Between Genealogy and Epistemology: Psychology, Politics, and Knowledge in the Thought of Michel Foucault* (University Park: Pennsylvania State University Press, 1993), 43.

48. Michel Foucault, *Society Must Be Defended: Lectures at the Collège de France, 1975–1976,* ed. François Ewald, Alessandro Fontana, and Mauro Bertani, trans. David Macey (New York: Picador, 2003 [1976]), 243.

49. Foucault, *The History of Sexuality,* 138.

50. Ibid., 141.

51. Foucault, *Society Must Be Defended.*

52. Ibid., 266.

53. Biological theories of race, produced as part of the disciplinary knowledges of biopower, were mobilized to rationalize the expansionism and exploitation that accompanied colonialism and slavery. As I discussed in the critical race theory framework, scientific racism operated by deploying scientific justifications for racial conquest and domination.

54. Foucault, *Society Must Be Defended,* 258.

55. For more on the links between biological theory, eugenics, and race, see Duster, *Backdoor to Eugenics*; Graves, *The Emperor's New Clothes*; Paul, *The Politics of Heredity*; Peter Weingart, "The Thin Line between Eugenics and Preventive Medicine," in *Identity and Intolerance: Nationalism, Racism, and Xenophobia in Germany and the United States,* ed. Norbert Finzsch and Deitmar Schirmer (Cambridge: Cambridge University Press, 1998), 397–412; Zuberi, *Thicker Than Blood.*

56. Jackie Orr, *Panic Diaries: A Genealogy of Panic Disorder* (Durham, N.C.: Duke University Press, 2006), 11.

57. Melbourne Tapper, *In the Blood: Sickle Cell Anemia and the Politics of Race* (Philadelphia: University of Pennsylvania Press, 1999).

2. The Emergence of Metabolic Syndrome

1. The analysis of emergence situates the emergence of a practice or discourse within a broader network of institutionally based power/knowledge relationships. For more on the genealogical analysis of emergence, reference my discussion in chapter 1.

2. I have selected the year 1956 as a way to mark the publication of the research of Jean Vague, a French physician whose work on metabolism is considered by many metabolic syndrome scientists to be foundational to the new field. I discuss Dr. Vague's work at several points throughout the chapter.

3. Jean Vague, "The Degree of Masculine Differentiation of Obesities: A Factor Determining Predisposition to Diabetes, Atherosclerosis, Gout and Uric Calculous Disease," *American Journal of Clinical Nutrition* 4 (1956): 20.

4. Researchers at the Metabolic Syndrome Institute, a Web-based organization of biomedical researchers whose primary goal is to promulgate the idea of the metabolic syndrome, attribute the concept to Dr. Vague. Several prominent metabolic syndrome researchers belong to this group, including Dr. Scott Grundy (http://www.metabolic-syndrome-institute.org/medical_information/history/#lien_a) (accessed December 20, 2006). Indeed, many others note the centrality of Dr. Vague's thought, but rarely do they explore his paper, which I do here. See Jean Vague, "La différenciation sexuelle, facteur déterminant des formes de l'obésité," *Presse Medicine* 30 (1947): 39; Vague, "The Degree of Masculine Differentiation of Obesities," 20–34.

5. Vague, "The Degree of Masculine Differentiation of Obesities," 21. Subsequent references are given in the text.

6. Ibid., 31. The islet of Langerhans is a part of the pancreas that is responsible for insulin production.

7. Karl Hitzenberger, "Über den Blutruck bei Diabetes Mellitus," *Weiner Arch Innere Med* 2 (1922): 461–66; E. Kylin, "Studien über das Hypertonie-Hyperglykemie-Hypoerurikemie Syndrome," *Zentrablatt für Innere Medizin* 7 (1923): 105–27; G. Maranon, "Über Hyperonie und Zuckerkrankheit," *Zentrablatt für Innere Medizin* 43 (1922): 169–76.

8. H. P. Himsworth, "Diabetes Mellitus: A Differentiation into Insulin-Sensitive and Insulin-Insensitive Types," *Lancet* 1 (1936): 127–30.

9. William B. Kannel, Daniel McGee, and Tavia Gordon, "A General Cardiovascular Risk Profile: The Framingham Study," *The American Journal of Cardiology* 38 (1976): 46–51. For a detailed accounting of the Framingham study and its approach to race and heart health, see Anne Pollock's *Medicating Race: Heart Disease and Durable Preoccupations with Difference* (Durham, N.C.: Duke University Press, 2012). The National Heart Institute is the institutional precursor to the National Heart, Lung, and Blood Institute (NHLBI) of the National Institutes of Health (NIH).

10. www.cdc.gov/nchs/about/major/nhis/hisdesc.htm (accessed October 23, 2006).

11. See my discussion of these population heart studies later in this section.

12. John M. Last, *A Dictionary of Epidemiology* (Oxford: Oxford University Press, 1995).

13. K. G. Alberti, P. Zimmet, and J. Shaw, "Metabolic Syndrome—A New Worldwide Definition: A Consensus Statement from the International Diabetes Federation," *Diabetes Medicine* 23 (2006): 473.

14. http://www2.merriam-webster.com/cgi-bin/mwmednlm (accessed March 5, 2009).

15. J. P. Camus, "Gout, Diabetes, and Hyperlipidemia: A Metabolic Trisyndrome," *Rev Rhum Mal Osteoartic* 33 (1966): 10–14.

16. P. Avogaro, G. Crepaldi, G. Enzi, et al., "Associazione di iperlipidemia, diabete mellito e obesita di medio grado," *Acta Diabetol Lat* 4 (1967): 36–41. In 1993, this construct gets revived in a book edited by Crepaldi, *Diabetes, Obesity, and Hyperlipidemia: The Plurimetabolic Syndrome*, ed. G. Crepaldi, A. Tiengo, and E. Manzato (Amsterdam: Elsevier Science, 1993).

17. Hellmut Mehnert and H. Kuhlmann, "Hypertonie und Diabetes Mellitus," *Deutsches Medizinisches Journal* 19 (1968): 567–71.

18. G. B. Phillips, "Relationship between Serum Sex-Hormones and Glucose, Insulin, and Lipid Abnormalities in Men with Myocardial-Infarction," *Proceedings of the National Academy of Sciences of the United States of America* 74 (1977): 1729–33; G. B. Phillips, "Sex Hormones, Risk Factors and Cardiovascular Disease," *American Journal of Medicine* 65 (1978): 7–11; G. B. Phillips, T. J. Jing, and S. B. Heymsfield, "Relationships in Men of Sex Hormones, Insulin, Adiposity, and Risk Factors for Myocardial Infarction," *Metabolism* 52 (2003): 784–90.

19. H. Haller, "Epidemiology and Associated Risk Factors of Hyperlipoproteinemia," *Z Gesamte Inn Med* 32 (1977): 124–28; P. Singer, "Diagnosis of Primary Hyperlipoproteinemias," *Z Gesamte Inn Med* 32 (1977): 129–33; V. E. Ziegler and J. T. Briggs, "Tricyclic Plasma Levels: Effect of Age, Race, Sex, and Smoking," *Journal of the American Medical Association* 14 (1977): 2167–69.

20. M. Hanefeld and W. Leonhardt, "Das Metabolische Syndrom (the Metabolic Syndrome)," *Dt Gesundh-Wesen* 36 (1981): 545–51.

21. Gerald M. Reaven, "Banting Lecture 1988: Role of Insulin Resistance in Human Disease," *Diabetes* 37 (1988): 1595–1607. The Banting Lecture is published annually in the journal *Diabetes,* the flagship journal of the American Diabetes Association. As of August 19, 2008, Reaven's published lecture had been cited 5,953 times.

22. In the 1980s, three groups of researchers created three new techniques for measuring insulin resistance. Ralph DeFronzo and colleagues developed the "euglycemic hyperinsulinemic clamp technique" in 1983, and it still is the DeFronzo gold-standard procedure to measure insulin resistance (see Ralph A. DeFronzo, Eleuterio Ferrannini, and Veikko Koivisto, "New Concepts in the Pathogenesis and Treatment of Noninsulin-Dependent Diabetes Mellitus," *American Journal of Medicine* 74 [1983]: 52–81). Other noteworthy techniques include the "homeostasis model assessment-insulin resistance index" (D. R. Matthews, J. P. Hosker, A. S. Rudenski, B. A. Naylor, D. F. Treacher, and R.C. Turner, "Homeostasis Model Assessment: Insulin Resistance and Beta-cell Function from Fasting Plasma Glucose and Insulin Concentrations in Man," *Diabetologia* 28 [1985]: 412–19) and the "oral glucose tolerance test" (Francesco Belfiore, Silvia Iannello, and Giovanni Volpicelli, "Insulin Sensitivity Indices Calculated from Basal and OGTT-Induced Insulin, Glucose, and FFA Levels," *Molecular Genetics and Metabolism* 63 [1998]: 134–41).

23. Gerald M. Reaven, "Bantling Lecture 1988: Role of Insulin Resistance in Human Disease," *Diabetes* 37 (1988): 1605.

24. Gerald Reaven, Terry Kristen Strom, and Barry Fox, *Syndrome X: The Silent Killer: The New Heart Disease Risk* (New York: Simon & Schuster, 2000).

25. In this simple schema, three points are awarded if your fasting glucose is greater than 11, or your glucose at two hours into the Glucose Tolerance Test is greater than 140; fasting triglyceride level is greater than 200; fasting HDL-cholesterol level is lower than 35; blood pressure is greater than 145/90. You earn one point if your weight check reveals that you are more than fifteen pounds overweight; your family has a history of heart disease, high blood pressure (hypertension), or diabetes; your lifestyle is characterized by physical inactivity in both work and leisure hours. Your risk of having a heart attack triggered by syndrome X can be low (0–4 points), moderate (5–8 points), high (9–12), or very high (13 or more) (adapted from ibid., 68).

26. N. M. Kaplan, "The Deadly Quartet: Upper-Body Obesity, Glucose Intolerance, Hypertriglyceridemia, and Hypertension," *Archives of Internal Medicine* 149 (1989): 1514–20; DeFronzo, Ferrannini, and Koivisto, "New Concepts in the Pathogenesis and Treatment of Noninsulin-Dependent Diabetes Mellitus," 52–81; R. DeFronzo and E. Ferrannini, "Insulin Resistance: A Multifaceted Syndrome Responsible for NIDDM," *Diabetes Care* 14 (1991): 173–94; I. Hjermann, "The Metabolic Cardiovascular Syndrome: Syndrome X, Reaven's Syndrome, Insulin Resistance Syndrome, Atherothrombogenic Syndrome," *Journal of Cardiovascular Pharmacology* 24 (1992): 461–64; P. Z. Zimmet, V. R. Collins, G. K. Dowse, K. G. M. Alberti, J. Tuomilehto, L. T. Knight, H. Gareeboo, P. Chitson, and D. Fareed, "Is Hyperinsulinemia a Central Characteristic of a Chronic Cardiovascular Risk Factor Clustering Syndrome—Mixed Findings in Asian Indian, Creole and Chinese Mauritians," *Diabetic Medicine* 11 (1994): 388–96; Angela D. Liese, Elizabeth J. Mayer-Davis, and Steven M. Haffner, "Development of Multiple Metabolic Syndrome: An Epidemiologic Perspective," *Epidemiologic Reviews* 20 (1998): 157–72.

27. http://www.cdc.gov/nchs/data/icd/icdp0500.pdf (accessed February 10, 2009).

28. http://www.icd9data.com/2009/Volume1/240–279/270–279/277/277.7.htm (accessed February 11, 2009).

29. National Cholesterol Education Program, "Executive Summary of the Third Report of the National Cholesterol Education Program (NCEP) Expert Panel on Detection, Evaluation, and Treatment of High Blood Cholesterol in Adults (Adult Treatment Panel III)," *Journal of the American Medical Association* 285 (2001): 2486–97.

30. National Institutes of Health, "The Metabolic Syndrome," in *Diabetes Mellitus Interagency Coordinating Committee Meeting* (Bethesda, Md.: National Institutes of Health, 2003), 9.

31. Daniel Einhorn, Gerald Reaven, R. H. Cobin, Earl S. Ford, O. P. Ganda, Y. Handelsman, R. Hellman, P. S. Jellinger, D. Kendall, R. M. Krauss, N. D. Neufeld, S. M. Petak, H. W. Rodbard, J. A. Seibel, D. A. Smith, and P. W. Wilson, "American College of Endocrinology Position Statement on the Insulin Resistance Syndrome," *Endocrinology Practice* 9 (2003): 236–52.

32. Gerald Reaven, "Syndrome X: 10 Years After," *Drugs* 58 (1999): 19; Gerald Reaven, "The Metabolic Syndrome or the Insulin Resistance Syndrome? Different Names, Different Concepts, and Different Goals," *Endocrinology and Metabolism Clinics of North America* 33 (2004): 283; Gerald M. Reaven, "Insulin Resistance, Cardiovascular Disease, and the Metabolic Syndrome," *Diabetes Care* 27 (2004): 1011; Gerald M. Reaven, "Dr. Reaven Responds," *Clinical Chemistry* 51 (2005): 1083; Gerald M. Reaven, "The Metabolic Syndrome: Requiescat in Pace," *Clinical Chemistry* 51 (2005): 931.

33. I discuss AstraZeneca again in chapter 4 because it is the producer of Crestor, a cholesterol-lowering medication that has been studied in populations classified with the metabolic syndrome.

34. Alberti et al., "Metabolic Syndrome—A New Worldwide Definition," 269–480.

35. The proinflammatory state refers to elevated levels of C-reactive protein, another biochemical that has been associated with metabolic syndrome.

36. Scott M. Grundy, James I. Cleeman, Stephen R. Daniels, Karen A. Donato, Robert H. Eckel, Barry A. Franklin, David J. Gordon, Ronald M. Krauss, Peter J. Savage, Sidney C. Smith Jr., John A. Spertus, and Fernando Costa, "Diagnosis and Management of the Metabolic Syndrome: An American Heart Association/ National Heart, Lung, and Blood Institute Executive Summary Scientific Statement," *Circulation* 112 (2005): 2735–52.

37. Ibid., 2736.

38. Ibid., 2737.

39. Ibid., 2745.

40. R. Kahn, J. Buse, E. Ferrannini, and M. Stern, "The Metabolic Syndrome: Time for a Critical Appraisal: Joint Statement from the American Diabetes Association and the European Association for the Study of Diabetes," *Diabetes Care* 28 (2005): 2289–2304.

41. Ibid., 2299.

42. The eight reasons are the following: (1) the criteria for metabolic syndrome are ambiguous or incomplete and the rationale for threshold values of specific biomarkers are ill-defined; (2) the value of including diabetes in the definition is questionable; (3) insulin resistance as the unifying etiology of metabolic syndrome is unclear; (4) there is no clear basis for including or excluding other cardiovascular disease (CVD) risk factors; (5) cardiovascular risk value is variable and dependent on the specific risk factors present; (6) the CVD risk associated with

the syndrome appears to be no greater than the sum of its parts; (7) treatment of the syndrome is no different than the treatment for each of its components; and (8) the medical value of diagnosing the syndrome is unclear.

43. Kahn et al., "The Metabolic Syndrome," 2291. See chapter 3 for more analysis of this racial conceptualization.

3. The Scientific Racism of Metabolism

1. http://www.nhlbi.nih.gov/health/health-topics/topics/ms/ (accessed September 20, 2014; emphasis added).

2. http://diabetes.niddk.nih.gov/dm/pubs/insulinresistance/#metabolic (accessed September 20, 2014; emphasis added). It is important to note that the NIDDK says that insulin resistance syndrome and metabolic syndrome are the same thing.

3. Stephen Jay Gould, *The Mismeasure of Man*, 2d ed. (New York: W. W. Norton, 1996); Nancy L. Stepan, *The Idea of Race in Science: Great Britain 1800–1960* (London: MacMillan, 1982); George W. Stocking, *Race, Culture, and Evolution: Essays in the History of Anthropology* (Chicago: University of Chicago Press, 1968); Warwick Anderson, *Colonial Pathologies: American Tropical Medicine, Race, and Hygiene in the Philippines* (Durham, N.C.: Duke University Press, 2006); Edwin Black, *War against the Weak: Eugenics and America's Campaign to Create a Master Race* (New York: Four Walls Eight Windows Press, 2003).

4. Elazar Barkan, *The Retreat of Scientific Racism: Changing Concepts of Race in Britain and the United States between the World Wars* (New York: Cambridge University Press, 1992); Daniel Kevles, *In the Name of Eugenics: Genetics and the Uses of Heredity* (Cambridge: Harvard University Press, 1985); Stepan, *The Idea of Race in Science: Great Britain 1800–1960*.

5. David Theo Goldberg, *The Racial State* (Malden, Mass.: Blackwell Publishers, 2002), 94.

6. Zygmunt Bauman, *Modernity and the Holocaust* (Ithaca, N.Y.: Cornell University Press, 1989).

7. Ann Morning, *The Nature of Race: How Scientists Think and Teach about Human Difference* (Berkeley: University of California Press, 2011).

8. United Nations Educational, Scientific and Cultural Organization, *The Race Question*, vol. 3 (Paris: United Nations Educational, Scientific and Cultural Organization, 1950), 5.

9. Paolo Palladino and Michael Worboys, "Science and Imperialism," *Isis* 84 (1993): 91–102; Craig S. Wilder, *Ebony and Ivy: Race, Slavery, and the Troubled History of America's Universities* (New York: Bloomsbury Press, 2013); Ashley Montagu, *Man's Most Dangerous Myth: The Fallacy of Race* (New York: Oxford University Press, 1974); Audrey Smedley and Brian Smedley, "Race as Biology Is Fiction, Racism as a Social Problem Is Real," *American Psychologist* 60(1) (2005): 16–26.

10. Harriet A. Washington, *Medical Apartheid: The Dark History of Medical Experimentation on Black Americans from Colonial Times to the Present* (New York: Doubleday, 2006).

11. Daniel Kevles, *In the Name of Eugenics: Genetics and the Uses of Heredity* (Cambridge: Harvard University Press, 1985); Diane B. Paul, *The Politics of Heredity: Essays on Eugenics, Biomedicine, and the Nature–Nurture Debate* (Albany: State University of New York Press, 1998); Tukufu Zuberi, *Thicker Than Blood: How Racial Statistics Lie* (Minneapolis: University of Minnesota Press, 2001).

12. Karl Hitzenberger, "Über den Blutruck bei Diabetes Mellitus," *Weiner Arch Innere Med* 2 (1922): 461–66; E. Kylin, "Studien über das Hypertonie-Hyperglykemie-Hypoerurikemie Syndrome," *Zentralblatt für Innere Medizin* 7 (1923): 105–27; G. Maranon, "Über Hyperonie und Zuckerkrankheit," *Zentralblatt für Innere Medizin* 43 (1922): 169–76; Jean Vague, "The Degree of Masculine Differentiation of Obesities: A Factor Determining Predisposition to Diabetes, Atherosclerosis, Gout and Uric Calculous Disease," *American Journal of Clinical Nutrition* 4 (1956).

13. Christopher Crenner, "Race and Laboratory Norms: The Critical Insights of Julian Herman Lewis (1891–1989)," *Isis* 105 (2014): 477–507; Steven Epstein, "Bodily Differences and Collective Identities: The Politics of Gender and Race in Biomedical Research in the United States," *Body and Society* 10 (2004): 183–203; Veronika Lipphardt and Jörg Niewöhner, "Producing Difference in an Age of Biosociality: Biohistorical Narratives, Standardisation, and Resistance as Translations," *Science, Technology, and Innovation Studies* 3 (2007): 45–65.

14. David R. Williams and Chaquita Collins, "US Socioeconomic and Racial Differences in Health: Patterns and Explanations," *Annual Review of Sociology* 21 (1995): 349–86.

15. Steven Epstein, *Inclusion: The Politics of Difference in Medical Research* (Chicago: University of Chicago Press, 2007).

16. Several other studies illustrate the general argument presented here. See, for example, MESA (Multiethnic Study of Atherosclerosis)—D. E. Bild, D. A. Bluemke, G. L. Burke, R. Detrano, A. V. Diez Roux, A. R. Folsom, P. Greenland, D. R. Jacobs Jr., R. Kronmal, K. Liu, J. C. Nelson, D. O'Leary, M. F. Saad, S. Shea, M. Szklo, and R. P. Tracy, "Multi-Ethnic Study of Atherosclerosis: Objectives and Design," *American Journal of Epidemiology* 156(9) (2002): 871–81; IRAS (Insulin Resistance and Atherosclerosis Study)—A. Festa, R. D'Agostino Jr., G. Howard, L. Mykkanen, R. P. Tracy, and S. M. Haffner, "Chronic Subclinical Inflammation as Part of the Insulin Resistance Syndrome: The Insulin Resistance Atherosclerosis Study (IRAS)," *Circulation* 102(1) (2000): 42–47.

17. Lytt Gardner, Michael Stern, Steven Haffner, Sharon Gaskill, Helen Hazuda, John Relethford, and Clatyon Eifler, "Prevalence of Diabetes in Mexican Americans: Relationship to Percent of Gene Pool Dervied from Native American Sources," *Diabetes* 33(1) (1984): 86–92.

18. I will discuss the theory of genetic admixture in greater detail in the following section. However, it is important to mention that the focus on Native American admixture is commonplace given the exceptionally high rates of insulin-resistant diabetes in some Native American populations, such as the Pima.

19. www.clinicaltrials.gov/ct/show/NCT00005146 (accessed February 13, 2009). See E. Ferrannini, S. M. Haffner, B. D. Mitchell, and M. P. Stern, "Hyperinsulinaemia: The Key Feature of a Cardiovascular and Metabolic Syndrome," *Diabetologia* 34(6) (1991): 416–22; T. S. Han, N. Sattar, K. Williams, C. Gonzalez-Villalpando, M. E. Lean, and S. M. Haffner, "Prospective Study of C-reactive Protein in Relation to the Development of Diabetes and Metabolic Syndrome in the Mexico City Diabetes Study," *Diabetes Care* 25(11) (2002): 2016–21; J. B. Meigs, K. Williams L. M. Sullivan, K. J. Hunt, S. M. Haffner, M. P. Stern, C. Gonzalez-Villalpando, J. S. Perhanidis, D. M. Nathan, R. B. D'Agostino Jr., R. B. D'Agostino Sr., and P. W. Wilson, "Using Metabolic Syndrome Traits for Efficient Detection of Impaired Glucose Tolerance," *Diabetes Care* 27(6) (2004): 1417–26.

20. G. H. Hughes, G. Cutter, R. Donahue, G. D. Friedman, S. Hulley, E. Hunkeler, D. R. Jacobs, K. Liu, S. Orden, P. Pirie, B. Tucker, and L. Wagenknecht, "Recruitment in the Coronary-Artery Disease Risk Development in Young-Adults (Cardia) Study," *Controlled Clinical Trials* 8(4) (1987): S68–S73.

21. http://www.cardia.dopm.uab.edu/lad_info.htm (accessed February 16, 2009).

22. N. Krieger and S. Sidney, "Racial Discrimination and Blood Pressure: The CARDIA Study of Young Black and White Adults," *American Journal of Public Health* 86(10) (1998): 1370–78; M. A. Pereira, D. R. Jacobs Jr., L. Van Horn, M. L. Slattery, A. I. Kartashov, and D. S. Ludwig, "Dairy Consumption, Obesity, and the Insulin Resistance Syndrome in Young Adults: The CARDIA Study," *Journal of the American Medical Association* 287(16) (2002): 2081–89.

23. W. Rathmann, E. Funkhouser, A. R. Dyer, and J. M. Roseman, "Relations of Hyperuricemia with the Various Components of the Insulin Resistance Syndrome in Young Black and White Adults: The CARDIA Study," *Annals of Epidemiology* 8(4) (1998): 250–61; W. Shen, M. Punyanitya, J. Chen, D. Gallagher, J. Albu, X. Pi-Sunyer, C. Lewis, C. Grunfeld, S. Heshka, and S. Heymsfield, "Waist Circumference Correlates with Metabolic Syndrome Indicators Better Than Percentage Fat," *Obesity* 14(4) (2004): 727–36; M. Carnethon, J. Hill, C. Loria, S. Sidney, P. Savage, and K. Liu, "Risk Factors for Developing the Metabolic Syndrome in Young Adults," *Diabetes Care* 27 (2004): 2707–15.

24. http://www.cscc.unc.edu/aric/ (accessed February 16, 2009).

25. M. I. Schmidt, B. B. Duncan, R. L. Watson, A. R. Sharrett, F. L. Brancati, and G. Heiss, "A Metabolic Syndrome in Whites and African-Americans: The Atherosclerosis Risk in Communities Baseline Study," *Diabetes Care* 19(5) (1996): 414–18.

26. A. Liese, E. J. Mayer-Davis, H. A. Tyroler, C. E. Davis, U. Keil, M. I. Schmidt,

F. L. Brancati, and G. Heiss, "Familial Components of the Multiple Metabolic Syndrome: The ARIC Study," *Diabetologia* 40 (1997): 963–70; Schmidt et al., "A Metabolic Syndrome in Whites and African-Americans," 414–18; A. D. Liese, E. J. Mayer-Davis, H. A. Tyroler, C. E. Davis, U. Keil, B. B. Duncan, and G. Heiss, "Development of the Multiple Metabolic Syndrome in the ARIC Cohort: Joint Contribution of Insulin, BMI, and WHR," *Annals of Epidemiology* 7 (1997): 407–16.

27. http://jhs.jsums.edu/jhsinfo/ (accessed February 16, 2009).

28. H. Taylor, J. Liu, G. T. Wilson, S. H. Golden, E. Crook, C. Brunson, M. Steffes, W. Johnson, and J. Sung, "Distinct Component Profiles and High Risk among African Americans with Metabolic Syndrome: The Jackson Heart Study," *Diabetes Care* 31(6) (2008): 1248–53.

29. http://www.nhlbi.nih.gov/about/jackson/2ndpg.htm (accessed February 16, 2009); C. M. Burchfiel, T. N. Skelton, M. E. Andrew, R. J. Garrison, D. K. Arnett, D. W. Jones, et al., "Metabolic Syndrome and Echocardiographic Left Ventricular Mass in Blacks: The Atherosclerosis Risk in Communities (ARIC) Study," *Circulation* 112(6) (2005): 819–27; H. Taylor et al., "Distinct Component Profiles and High Risk among African Americans with Metabolic Syndrome," 1248–53.

30. Gerald M. Reaven, "Banting Lecture 1988: Role of Insulin Resistance in Human Disease," *Diabetes* 37 (1988): 1595–1607. The Banting lecture is published annually in the journal *Diabetes,* the flagship journal of the American Diabetes Association. As of March 4, 2013, Reaven's published lecture had been cited 8,241 times.

31. S. W. Shen, G. M. Reaven, and J. W. Farquhar, "Comparison of Impedance to Insulin-Mediated Glucose Uptake in Normal Subjects and in Subjects with Latent Diabetes," *Journal of Clinical Investigation* 49(12) (1970): 2151–60; H. Ginsberg, G. Kimmerling, J. M. Olefsky, and G. M. Reaven, "Demonstration of Insulin Resistance in Untreated Adult Onset Diabetic Subjects with Fasting Hyperglycemia," *Journal of Clinical Investigation* 55(3) (1975): 454–61.

32. Shen, Reaven, and Farquhar, "Comparison of Impedance to Insulin-Mediated Glucose Uptake in Normal Subjects and in Subjects with Latent Diabetes," 2151.

33. Gerald Reaven, Terry Kristen Strom, and Barry Fox, *Syndrome X: The Silent Killer: The New Heart Disease Risk* (New York: Simon & Schuster, 2000), 20.

34. C. Bogardus, S. Lillioja, D. M. Mott, C. Hollenbeck, and G. Reaven, "Relationship between Degree of Obesity and Invivo Insulin Action in Man," *American Journal of Physiology* 248(3) (1985): E286–E291. According to an NIDDK Web site on the special role the Pima have played in government biomedical research on diabetes, "This cooperative search between the Pima Indians and the NIH began in 1963 when the NIDDK (then called the National Institute of Arthritis, Diabetes and Digestive and Kidney Diseases), made a survey of rheumatoid arthritis among the Pimas and the Blackfeet of Montana. They discovered an extremely high rate of diabetes among the Pima Indians. Two years later, the Institute, the

Indian Health Service, and the Pima community set out to find some answers to this mystery" (http://diabetes.niddk.nih.gov/dm/pubs/pima/pathfind/pathfind.htm; accessed February 16, 2009).

35. Reaven, Strom, and Fox, *Syndrome X, 57.*

36. S. Lillioja, D. M. Mott, J. K. Zawadzki, A. A. Young, W. G. H. Abbott, W. C. Knowler, P. H. Bennett , P. Moll, and C. Bogardus, "Invivo Insulin Action Is Familial Characteristic in Nondiabetic Pima-Indians," *Diabetes* 36(11) (1987): 1329–35.

37. Reaven, Strom, and Fox, *Syndrome X, 57.*

38. Ibid., 58.

39. World Health Organization, *Obesity: Preventing and Managing the Global Epidemic* (Geneva: World Health Organization, 1997); World Health Organization, "Appropriate Body-Mass Index for Asian Populations and Its Implications for Policy and Intervention Strategies," *Lancet* 363 (2004): 157–63.

40. D. Einhorn, "American College of Endocrinology Position Statement on the Insulin Resistance Syndrome," *Endocrine Practice* 9(3) (2003): 236–39.

41. K. Alberti, P. Zimmet, and J. Shaw, "Metabolic Syndrome—A New Worldwide Definition: A Consensus Statement from the International Diabetes Federation," *Diabetes Medicine* 23(5) (2006): 473.

42. Ibid., 476.

43. D. Banerjee and A. Misra, "Does Using Ethnic Specific Criteria Improve the Usefulness of the Term Metabolic Syndrome? Controversies and Suggestions," *International Journal of Obesity* 31 (2007): 1340–49; N. Unwin, R. Bhopal, L. Hayes, M. White, S. Patel, D. Ragoobirsingh, and G. Alberti, "A Comparison of the New International Diabetes Federation Definition of Metabolic Syndrome to WHO and NCEP Definitions in Chinese, European and South Asian Origin Adults," *Ethnicity and Disease* 17 (summer 2007): 522–28.

44. S. Zhu, S. B. Heymsfield, H. Toyoshima, A. Wang, A. Pietrobelli, and S. Heshka, "Race-Ethnicity-Specific Waist Circumference Cutoffs for Identifying Cardiovascular Risk Factors," *American Journal of Clinical Nutrition* 81 (2005): 409–15; M. C. Desilets, D. Garrel, C. Couillard, A. Tremblay, J. P. Despres, C. Bouchard, and H. Delisle, "Ethnic Differences in Body Composition and Other Markers of Cardiovascular Disease Risk: Study in Matched Haitian and White Subjects from Quebec," *Obesity* 14(6) (2006): 1019–27; P. Bovet, D. Faeh, A. Gabriel, and L. Tappy, "The Prediction of Insulin Resistance with Serum Triglyceride and High-Density Lipoprotein Cholesterol Levels in an East African Population," *Archives of Internal Medicine* 166(11) (2006): 1236–37; A. E. Sumner and C. C. Cowie, "Ethnic Differences in the Ability of Triglyceride Levels to Identify Insulin Resistance," *Atherosclerosis* 196 (2008): 696–703; A. E. Sumner, K. B. Finley, D. J. Genovese, M. H. Criqui, and R. C. Boston, "Fasting Triglyceride and the Triglyceride-HDL Cholesterol Ratio Are Not Markers of Insulin Resistance

in African Americans," *Archives of Internal Medicine* 165(12) (2005): 1395–1400; P. Amarenco, P. Labreuche, and P.-J. Touboul, "High-Density Lipoprotein-Cholesterol and Risk of Stroke and Carotid Atherosclerosis: A Systematic Review," *Atherosclerosis* 196 (2008): 489–96.

45. L. T. Clark and F. El-Atat, "Metabolic Syndrome in African Americans: Implications for Preventing Coronary Heart Disease," *Clinical Cardiology* 30(4) (2007): 161–64; K. Ferdinand, L. Clark, K. Watson, R. Neal, C. Brown, B. Kong, B. Barnes, W. Cox, F. Zieve, J. Ycas, P. Sager, and A. Gold, "Comparison of Efficacy and Safety of Rosuvastatin versus Atorvastatin in African-American Patients in a Six-Week Randomized Trial," *American Journal of Cardiology* 97(2) (2006): 229–35; S. M. Grundy, J. I. Cleeman, C. N. B. Merz, H. B. Brewer Jr., L. T. Clark, D. B. Hunninghake, R. C. Pasternak, S. C. Smith Jr., and N. J. Stone, "Implications of Recent Clinical Trials for the National Cholesterol Education Program Adult Treatment Panel III Guidelines," *Circulation* 110(2) (2004): 227–39; S. C. Smith, S. R. Daniels, M. A. Quinones, S. K. Kumanyika, L. T. Clark, R. S. Cooper, E. Saunders, E. Ofili, and E. J. Sanchez, "Discovering the Full Spectrum of Cardiovascular Disease: Minority Health Summit 2003: Report of the Obesity, Metabolic Syndrome, and Hypertension Writing Group," *Circulation* 111(10) (2005): e134–e139.

46. W. Dallas Hall, Luther T. Clark, Nanette K. Wenger, Jackson T. Wright, Shiriki K. Kumankya, and Karol Watson, "The Metabolic Syndrome in African Americans: A Review," *Ethnicity & Disease* 13(4) (2003): 415. Recall that the San Antonio Heart Study was also designed to assess the degree of genetic admixture.

47. E. S. Tull and J. M. Roseman, "Diabetes in African Americans," in *Diabetes in America,* 2d ed. (Bethesda, Md.: National Institutes of Health, NIDDK National Diabetes Data Group, 1995), 614.

48. Hall et al., "The Metabolic Syndrome in African Americans," 415.

49. Duana Fullwiley, "The Biologistical Construction of Race: 'Admixture' Technology and the New Genetic Medicine," *Social Studies of Science* 38 (2008): 695–735.

50. Joan. H. Fujimura and Ramya Rajagopalan, "Different Differences: The Use of 'Genetic Ancestry' versus Race in Biomedical Human Genetic Research," *Social Studies of Science* 41 (2011): 15–30.

4. Killer Applications

1. Neil J. Stone, Jennifer Robinson, Alice H. Lichenstein, C. Noel Bairey Merz, Conrad B. Blum, Robert H. Eckel, Anne C. Goldberg, David Gordon, Daniel Levy, Donald M. Lloyd-Jones, Patrick McBridge, J. Stanford Schwartz, Susan T. Shero, Sidney C. Smith, Karol Watson, and Peter W. F. Wilson, "2013 ACC/AHA Guideline on the Treatment of Blood Cholesterol to Reduce Atherosclerotic Cardiovascular Risk in Adults: A Report of the American College of Cardiology/American

Heart Association Task Force on Practice Guidelines," *Circulation* (online version printed November 12, 2013).

2. Recall from chapter 1 that the analysis of descent traces the multiple sites of knowledge production by documenting the actual research instruments, procedures, and practices used in the study of the body.

3. Jonathan Kahn, *Race in a Bottle: The Story of BiDil and Racialized Medicine in a Post-Genomic Age* (New York: Columbia University Press, 2013).

4. There are other candidate drugs that could be examined here as well. Metabolic syndrome is increasingly used to refer to new drug targets, or new laboratory markers that reflect the efficacy of drug therapies. See Dario Giugliano, Antonio Ceriello, and Katherine Esposito, "Are There Specific Treatments for the Metabolic Syndrome?" *American Journal of Clinical Nutrition* 87 (2008): 8–11; Scott M. Grundy, James I. Cleeman, C. Noel Bairey Merz, H. Bryan Brewer Jr., Luther T. Clark, Donald B. Hunninghake, Richard C. Pasternak, Sidney C. Smith Jr., and Neil J. Stone, "Implications of Recent Clinical Trials for the National Cholesterol Education Program Adult Treatment Panel III Guidelines," *Circulation* 110 (2004): 227–39; Scott M. T. Grundy, "Drug Therapy of the Metabolic Syndrome Minimizing the Emerging Crisis in Polypharmacy," *Nature Reviews Drug Discovery* 5 (2006): 295–315; T. A. Jacobson, C. C. Case, S. Roberts, A. Buckley, K. M. Murtaugh, J. C. Y. Sung, D. Gause, C. Varas, and C. M. Ballantyne, "Characteristics of U.S. Adults with the Metabolic Syndrome and Therapeutic Implications," *Diabetes, Obesity and Metabolism* 6 (2004): 353; and Lawrence J. Lesko and A. J. Atkinson Jr., "Use of Biomarkers in Development, Surrogate Endpoints in Drug Regulatory Decision Making: Criteria, Validation Strategies," *Annual Review of Pharmacology & Toxicology* 41 (2001): 347–66.

5. *Oxford English Dictionary,* entry for "Killer Applications" (accessed online September 1, 2014).

6. Donna J. Haraway, *Modest_Witness@Second_Millennium. FemaleMan_Meets_OncoMouse* (New York: Routledge, 1997). Haraway uses the term "killer applications" in the following manner: "Software sufficiently powerful to revolutionize how computers are used—that is, how further hybrids of human and nonhumans take shape and act—are, unfortunately, called, killer applications. Comparable only to the importance of the word-processor and spreadsheet software, Mosaic-like browsers are likely to be such 'killer applications' that reconfigure practice in an immense array of domains. Mosaic was about the power to make hypertext and hypergraphic connections of the sort that produce the global subject of technoscience as a potent form of historical, contingent, specific human nature at the end of the millennium. Contesting how such subjects and hybrids are put together and taken apart is a critical feminist technoscientific practice" (126).

7. Larry Downes and Chunka Mui, *Unleashing the Killer App* (Cambridge: Harvard Business School Press, 1998), 4.

8. Saul Malozowski, "Comparative Efficacy: What We Know, What We Need to Know, and How We Can Get There," *Annals of Internal Medicine* 148 (2008): 702–3.

9. #1: Lipitor for cholesterol—74.8 million prescriptions; #4: Norvasc for hypertension and angina—38.3 million prescriptions; #5: Toprol-XL for hypertension—35 million; #7: Zocor for hypertension—29.6 million.

10. http://www.firstwordpharma.com/node/1096220#axzz2iN3I9KHx (accessed October 21, 2013). The other five metabolic drugs were #2: Plavix (9.92 billion), #9: Crestor (6.62 billion), #10: Lantus (6.38 billion), #14: Diovan (6.05 billion), and #17: Zocor (5.5445 billion).

11. David S. Jones and Roy H. Perlis, "Pharmacogenetics, Race, and Psychiatry," *Harvard Review of Psychiatry* 14 (2006); Kahn, *Race in a Bottle*; John A. Lynch and Tasha Dubriwny, "Drugs and Double Binds: Racial Identity and Pharmacogenomics in a System of Binary Race Logic," *Health Communication* 19(1) (2006): 61–73.

12. Troy Duster, "Race and Reification in Science," *Science* 307 (2005): 1050–51.

13. Ibid., 1050.

14. Lisa Gannett, "Group Categories in Pharmacogenetics Research," *Philosophy of Science* 72 (2005): 1232–47.

15. Ibid., 1235.

16. The case of antiretroviral drugs that treat HIV infection could also have been analyzed here. Many HIV drugs have metabolic side effects and metabolic syndrome is also being deployed to describe these effects. See C. Hadigan, J. B. Meigs, C. Corcoran, P. Rietschel, S. Piecuch, N. Basgoz, B. Davis, P. Sax, T. Stanley, P. W. F. Wilson, R. B. D'Agostino, and S. Grinspoon, "Metabolic Abnormalities and Cardiovascular Disease Risk Factors in Adults with Human Immunodeficiency Virus Infection and Lipodystrophy," *Clinical Infectious Diseases* 32 (2001): 130–39; H. P. Murata, W. Hruz, and M. Mueckler, "The Mechanism of Insulin Resistance Caused by HIV Protease Inhibitor Therapy," *Journal of Biological Chemistry* 275 (2000): 20251–54; and S. Safrin and C. Grunfeld, "Fat Distribution and Metabolic Changes in Patients with HIV Infection," *Aids* 13 (1999): 2493–2505.

17. Michel Foucault, *Madness and Civilization: A History of Insanity in the Age of Reason,* trans. Richard Howard (New York: Vintage Books, 1965); Allan V. Horowitz, "The Sociological Study of Mental Illness: A Critique and Synthesis of Four Perspectives," in *Handbook of the Sociology of Mental Health,* 2d ed., ed. Carol. S. Anseshensel, Jo C. Phelan, and Alex Bierman (New York: Springer, 2013), 57–78.

18. Martha L. Bruce and Patrick Raue, "Mental Illness as Psychiatric Disorder," in Anseshensel, Phelan, and Bierman, *Handbook of the Sociology of Mental Health,* 41.

19. Ibid., 46.

20. S. J. Keith, D. A. Regier, and D. Rae, "Schizophrenic Disorders," in *Psychiatric Disorders in America,* ed. L. Robins and D. Reiger (New York: Free Press, 1991), 33–52.

21. V. R. Adebimpe, "White Norms and Psychiatric Diagnosis of Black Patients," *American Journal of Psychiatry* 138 (1981): 279–85; V. R. Adebimpe, "A Second Opinion on the Use of White Norms in Psychiatric Diagnosis of Black Patients," *Psychiatric Annals* 34 (2004): 542–51; V. R. Adebimpe, "Race, Racism, and Epidemiological Surveys," *Hospital and Community Psychiatry* 45 (1994): 27–31; V. R. Adebimpe, "Constraints on the Validity of Black/White Differences in Epidemiologic Measurements," *Journal of the National Medical Association* 95 (2003): 743–45; Paul E. Keck Jr., Lesley M. Arnold, Jacqueline Collins, Rodgers M. Wilson, David E. Fleck, Kimberly B. Corey, Jennifer Amicone, and Victor R. Adebimpe, "Ethnicity and Diagnosis in Patients with Affective Disorders," *Journal of Clinical Psychiatry* 64 (2003): 747–54; S. M. Strakowski, M. Flaum, and X. Amador, "Racial Differences in the Diagnosis of Psychosis," *Schizophrenia Research* 21 (1996): 117–24.

22. Gerald N. Grob, "The Origins of Psychiatric Epidemiology," *American Journal of Public Health* 75 (1985): 229–36.

23. George W. Dowdall, "Mental Hospitals and Deinstitutionalizations," in Aneshensel, Phelan, and Bierman, *Handbook of the Sociology of Mental Health,* 519–38.

24. Jonathan M. Metzl, *The Protest Psychosis: How Schizophrenia Became a Black Disease* (Boston: Beacon Press, 2011).

25. Pauline Agbayani-Siewart, David T. Takeuchi, and Rosavinia W. Pangan, "Mental Illness in a Multicultural Context," in Aneshensel, Phelan, and Bierman, *Handbook of the Sociology of Mental Health,* 19–36.

26. Carl I. Cohen and Leslie Marino, "Racial and Ethnic Differences in the Prevalence of Psychotic Symptoms in the General Population," *Psychiatric Services* 64(11) (2013): 1103–9; Robert C. Schwartz and David M. Blankenship, "Racial Disparities in Psychotic Disorder Diagnosis: A Review of Empirical Literature," *World Journal of Psychiatry* 4(4) (2014): 133–40.

27. David Herzberg, *Happy Pills in America: From Miltown to Prozac* (Baltimore: Johns Hopkins University Press, 2009).

28. H. Chung, J. C. Mahler, and T. Kakuma, "Racial Differences in Treatment of Psychiatric Inpatients," *Psychiatric Services* 46 (1995): 586–91; M. V. Rudorfer and E. Robins, "Amitriptyline Overdose—Clinical Effects on Tricyclic Antidepressant Plasma-Levels," *Journal of Clinical Psychiatry* 43 (1982): 457–60.

29. G. L. Daumit, R. M. Crum, E. Guallar, N. R. Powe, A. B. Primm, D. M. Steinwachs, and D. E. Ford, "Outpatient Prescriptions for Atypical Antipsychotics for African Americans, Hispanics, and Whites in the United States," *Archives of General Psychiatry* 60 (2003): 121.

30. J. P. McEvoy, P. Scheifler, and A. Francos, "An Expert Consensus Guideline Series Treatment of Schizophrenia," *Journal of Clinical Psychiatry* 60 (1999): 9–34.

31. Eugene Barrett, Lawrence Blonde, Steven Clement, John David, Klein Devlin, John M. Kane, Samuel Klein, and William Torrey, "Consensus Development Conference on Antipsychotic Drugs and Obesity and Diabetes," *Diabetes Care* 27 (2004): 596–601.

32. Representatives from the American Diabetes Association, the American Psychiatric Association, the American Association of Clinical Endocrinologists, the North American Association for the Study of Obesity, the Food and Drug Administration, AstraZeneca, Bristol-Myers Squibb, Janssen, Lilly, and Pfizer were present.

33. W. S. Fenton and M. R. Chavez, "Medication-Induced Weight Gain and Dyslipidemia in Patients with Schizophrenia," *American Journal of Psychiatry* 163 (2006): 1697–1704.

34. www.fda.gov/fsn (accessed August 22, 2008—Show #28, June 2004).

35. S. R. Marder, S. M. Essock, A. L. Miller, R. W. Buchanan, D. E. Casey, J. M. Davis, J. M. Kane, J. A. Lieberman, N. R. Schooler, N. Covell, S. Stroup, E. M. Weissman, D. A. Wirshing, C. S. Hall, L. Pogach, X. Pi-Sunyer, J. T. Bigger, A. Friedman, D. Kleinberg, S. J. Yevich, B. Davis, and S. Shon, "Physical Health Monitoring of Patients with Schizophrenia," *American Journal of Psychiatry* 161 (2004): 1334–49.

36. Barrett et al., "Consensus Development Conference on Antipsychotic Drugs and Obesity and Diabetes," 600.

37. B. R. Basson, B. J. Kinon, C. C. Taylor, K. A. Szymanski, J. A. Gilmore, and G. D. Tollefson, "Factors Influencing Acute Weight Change in Patients with Schizophrenia Treated with Olanzapine, Haloperidol, or Risperidone," *Journal of Clinical Psychiatry* 62 (2001): 231–38.

38. E. Kuno and A. B. Rothbard, "Racial Disparities in Antipsychotic Prescription Patterns for Patients with Schizophrenia," *American Journal of Psychiatry* 159 (2002): 567–72; S. P. Segel, J. R. Bola, and M. A. Watson, "Race, Quality of Care and Antipsychotic Prescribing Practices in Psychatric Emergency Services," *Psychiatric Services* 47 (1996): 282–86; J. T. Walkup, D. D. McAlpine, M. Olfson, L. E. Labay, C. Boyer, and S. Hansell, "Patients with Schizophrenia at Risk for Excessive Antipsychotic Dosing," *Journal of Clinical Psychiatry* 61 (2000): 344–48; S. W. Woods, M. C. Sullivan, E. C. Neuse, E. Diaz, C. B. Baker, S. H. Madonick, E. E. H. Griffith, and J. L. Steiner, "Racial and Ethnic Effects on Antipsychotic Prescribing Practices in a Community Mental Health Center," *Psychiatric Services* 54 (2003): 177–79.

39. G. L. Daumit, R. M. Crum, E. Guallar, N. R. Powe, A. B. Primm, D. M. Steinwachs, and D. E. Ford, "Outpatient Prescriptions for Atypical Antipsychotics for African Americans, Hispanics, and Whites in the United States," *Archives of General Psychiatry* 60 (2003): 121–28; D. M. Herbeck, J. C. West, I. Ruditis, F. F.

Duffy, D. J. Fitek, C. C. Bell, and L. R. Snowden, "Variations in Use of Second-Generation Antipsychotic Medication by Race among Adult Psychiatric Patients," *Psychiatric Services* 55 (2004): 677–84; T. L. Mark, R. Dirani, E. Slade, and P. A. Russo, "Access to New Medications to Treat Schizophrenia," *Journal of Behavioral Health Services and Research* 29 (2002): 15–29; P. S. Wang, J. C. West, T. Tanielian, and H. A. Pincus, "Recent Patterns and Predictors of Antipsychotic Medication Regimes Used to Treat Schizophrenia and Other Psychotic Disorders," *Schizophrenia Bulletin* 26 (2000): 451–55.

40. Office of the Surgeon General, *Mental Health: Culture, Race, and Ethnicity: A Supplement to Mental Health: A Report of the Surgeon General* (Rockville, Md.: Substance Abuse and Mental Health Services Administration, Center for Mental Health Services, 2001).

41. Ibid. The reports cited are V. E. Ziegler and J. T. Briggs, "Tricyclic Plasma Levels: Effect of Age, Race, Sex, and Smoking," *Journal of the American Medical Association* 14 (1977): 2167–69; M. V. Rudorfer and E. Robins, "Amitriptyline Overdose—Clinical Effects on Tricyclic Anti-Depressant Plasma-Levels," *Journal of Clinical Psychiatry* 43 (1982): 457–60; L. DiAnne Bradford, Andrea Gaedigk, and Steven Leeder, "High Frequency of CYP2D6 Poor and 'Intermediate' Metabolizers in Black Populations: A Review and Preliminary Data," *Psychopharmacology Bulletin* 34 (1998): 797–804.

42. Office of the Surgeon General, *Mental Health,* 67; emphasis added.

43. M. V. Relling, J. Cherrie, M. J. Schell, W. P. Petros, W. H. Meyer, and W. E. Evans, "Lower Prevalence of the Debrisoquin Oxidative Poor Metabolizer Phenotype in American Black versus White Subjects," *Clinical Pharmacology and Therapeutics* 50 (1991): 308–13.

44. Walkup et al., "Patients with Schizophrenia at Risk for Excessive Antipsychotic Dosing," 347.

45. Relling et al., "Lower Prevalence of the Debrisoquin Oxidative Poor Metabolizer Phenotype in American Black versus White Subjects," 346.

46. http://www.fda.gov/AboutFDA/WhatWeDo/History/ProductRegulation/SelectionsFromFDLIUpdateSeriesonFDAHistory/ucm082054.htm (accessed on January 4, 2009). The term "statins" refers to a class of drugs that are hydroxylmethl glutaryl coenzyme A (HMG CoA) reductase inhibitors. See Suzanna White Junod, "Statins: A Success Story Involving FDA, Academia, and Industry," *Update: A Bimonthly Publication of the FDA Law Institute* (2007).

47. Jeremy A. Greene, "Statins: The Abnormal and the Pathological: Cholesterol, Statins, and the Threshold of Disease," in *Medicating Modern America: Prescription Drugs in History,* ed. A. Tone and E. S. Watkins (New York: New York University Press, 2007), 183–228.

48. Junod, "Statins."

49. The first six statins in order of their FDA approval are Mevacor (lova-

statin), Lescol (fluvastatin), Lipitor (atoravastatin), Zocor (simvastatin), Prava-
chol (pravastatin), and Crestor (rosuvastatin).

50. See M. K. Ito, R. J. Cheung, E. K. Gupta, K. K. Birtcher, P. H. Chong, T. M.
Bianco, and B. E. Bleske, "Key Articles, Guidelines, and Consensus Papers Relative to the Treatment of Dyslipidemias—2005," *Pharmacotherapy* 26 (2006):
939–1010; National Cholesterol Education Program, "Executive Summary of
the Third Report of the National Cholesterol Education Program (NCEP) Expert Panel on Detection, Evaluation, and Treatment of High Blood Cholesterol in
Adults (Adult Treatment Panel III)," *Journal of the American Medical Association*
285 (2001): 2486–97.

51. Scott M. Grundy, H. Bryan Brewer Jr., James I. Cleeman, Sidney C. Smith
Jr., Claude Lenfant, and Participants for the Conference, "Definition of Metabolic
Syndrome: Report of the National Heart, Lung, and Blood Institute/American
Heart Association Conference on Scientific Issues Related to Definition," *Circula-
tion* 109 (2004): 433–38.

52. www.astrazeneca-us.com/modules/PRMS/display.asp?id-591959 (accessed
October 23, 2006). The Galaxy Program has included more than fifty thousand
research subjects in fifty nations.

53. The trials are (1) ARIES; (2) the STARSHIP Study (Study Assessing Rosuvastatin in Hispanic Population); and (3) The IRIS Study (Investigation of Rosuvastatin in South Asian Subjects). For (2), see R. Lloret, J. Ycas, M. Stein, and S. M.
Haffner, "Comparison of Rosuvastatin versus Atorvastin in Hispanic-Americans
with Hypercholesterolemia," *American Journal of Cardiology* 98 (2006): 768–73.

54. K. C. Ferdinand, L. T. Clark, K. E. Watson, R. C. Neal, C. D. Brown, B. W.
Kong, B. O. Barnes, W. R. Cox, F. J. Zieve, J. Ycas, P. T. Sager, and A. Gold, "Comparison of Efficacy and Safety of Rosuvastatin versus Atorvastatin in African-
American Patients in a Six-Week Randomized Trial," *American Journal of Cardiology* 97 (2006): 229–35.

55. Research subjects were recruited from the practices of physicians who participated in the study and all had been on either diet or drug therapy for high
cholesterol during the previous three months. The physician sample (n=401) was
drawn from a larger pool of practicing doctors who represented the top 26 percent of statin prescribers who worked under the auspices of IMS Health (based
in Westport, Connecticut). These doctors were responsible for 55 percent of prescriptions for lipid-lowering drugs in 2002 and may be what the authors call
"enthusiasts" who may manage lipids more aggressively than the average.

56. The investigators considered simvastatin and atoravastin "high-efficacy
statins."

57. Luther T. Clark, Kevin C. Maki, Ron Galant, David J. Maron, Thomas A.
Pearson, and Michael H. Davidson, "Ethnic Differences in Achievement of Cholesterol Treatment Goals," *Journal of General Internal Medicine* 21 (2006): 324;

T. A. Jacobson, M. M. Chin, C. L. Curry, V. Miller, V. Papademetriou, R. C. Schlant, and J. C. Larosa, "Efficacy and Safety of Pravastatin in African-Americans with Primary Hypercholesterolemia," *Archives of Internal Medicine* 155 (1995): 1900–1906.

58. H. Charles, C. B. Good, B. H. Hanusa, C. C. H. Chang, and J. Whittle, "Racial Differences in Adherence to Cardiac Medications," *Journal of the National Medical Association* 95 (2003): 17; P. H. Chong, P. J. Tzallas-Pontikes, J. D. Seeger, and T. D. Stamos, "The Low-Density Lipoprotein Cholesterol-Lowering Effect of Pravastatin and Factors Associated with Achieving Targeted Low-Density Lipoprotein Levels in an African-American Population," *Pharmacotherapy* 20 (2000): 1454–63; M. L. Williams, M. T. Morris, U. Ahmad, M. Youssef, W. Li, and N. Ertel, "Racial Differences in Compliance with NCEP II Recommendations for Secondary Prevention at a Veterans Affairs Medical Center," *Ethnicity & Disease* 12 (2002): 58–62.

59. Clark et al., "Ethnic Differences in Achievement of Cholesterol Treatment Goals," 324.

60. Ibid.

61. K. C. Ferdinand, "Dyslipidemia Treatment in African-Americans: Should Race Be a Factor?" *Future Lipidology* 1 (2006): 653–58; Jacobson et al., "Efficacy and Safety of Pravastatin in African-Americans with Primary Hypercholesterolemia," 1900–1906; J. C. LaRosa, W. Applegate, J. R. Crouse, D. B. Hunninghake, R. Grimm, R. Knopp, J. H. Eckfeldt, C. E. Davis, and D. J. Gordon, "Cholesterol-Lowering in the Elderly—Results of the Cholesterol Reduction in Seniors Program (Crisp) Pilot-Study," *Archives of Internal Medicine* 154 (1994): 529–39; L. M. Prisant, M. Downton, L. O. Watkins, H. Schnaper, R. H. Bradford, A. N. Chremos, and A. Langendorfer, "Efficacy and Tolerability of Lovastatin in 459 African-Americans with Hypercholesterolemia," *American Journal of Cardiology* 78 (1996): 420–24.

62. Clark et al., "Ethnic Differences in Achievement of Cholesterol Treatment Goals," 342.

63. L. T. Clark and F. El-Atat, "Metabolic Syndrome in African Americans: Implications for Preventing Coronary Heart Disease," *Clinical Cardiology* 30 (2007): 161–64.

64. Karol E. Watson, "Cardiovascular Risk Reduction among African Americans: A Call to Action," *Journal of the National Medical Association* 100 (2008): 18–26.

65. See Allhat Officers and Coordinators for the Allhat Collaborative Research Group, "Major Outcomes in High-Risk Hypertensive Patients Randomized to Angiotensin-Converting Enzyme Inhibitor or Calcium Channel Blocker vs Diuretic: The Antihypertensive and Lipid-Lowering Treatment to Prevent Heart Attack Trial (ALLHAT)," *Journal of the American Medical Association* 288 (2002):

2981–97; Joel A. Simon, Feng Lin, Stephen B. Hulley, Patricia J. Blanche, David Waters, Stephen Shiboski, Jerome I. Rotter, Deborah A. Nickerson, Huiying Yang, Mohammed Saad, and Ronald M. Krauss, "Phenotypic Predictors of Response to Simvastatin Therapy among African-Americans and Caucasians: The Cholesterol and Pharmacogenetics (CAP) Study," *American Journal of Cardiology* 97 (2006): 843–50.

66. Watson, "Cardiovascular Risk Reduction among African Americans," 22.

67. Ibid., 24; emphasis added.

68. D. G. Vidt, S. Harris, F. McTaggart, M. Ditmarsch, P. T. Sager, and J. M. Sorof, "Effect of Short-Term Rosuvastatin Treatment on Estimated Glomerular Filtration Rate," *American Journal of Cardiology* 97(11) (2006): 1602–6.

69. Watson, "Cardiovascular Risk Reduction among African Americans," 24.

70. Ibid.

71. Food and Drug Administration, *Guidance for Industry: Collection of Race and Ethnicity Data in Clinical Trials* (Rockville, Md.: U.S. Department of Health and Human Services, 2005). These FDA guidelines advocate the use of the Office of Management and Budget racial categories and were discussed in chapter 3.

72. Andrew Van Hook, *Sugar: Its Production, Technology, and Uses* (New York: Ronald Press Company, 1949), 129–30.

5. Sugar Stained with Blood

1. Jennifer Wenzel, Sharon W. Utz, Richard Steeves, Ivy Hinton, and Randy A. Jones, "'Plenty of Sickness': Descriptions by African Americans Living in Rural Areas with Type 2 Diabetes," *Diabetes Educator* 31(1) (2005): 98–107; John B. Schorling and J. Terry Saunders, "Is 'Sugar' the Same as Diabetes? A Community-Based Study among Rural African Americans," *Diabetes Care* 23(3) (2000): 330–34.

2. American Dietetic Association, "Evidence-Based Nutrition Principles and Recommendations for the Treatment and Prevention of Diabetes and Related Complications," *Diabetes Care* 26(supplement 1) (2003): S51–61; E. K. Caso, "Calculation of Diabetic Diets: Report of the Committee on Diabetic Diet Calculations, American Dietetic Association. Prepared Cooperatively with the Committee on Education, American Diabetes Association and Diabetes Branch, U.S. Public Health Service," *Journal of the American Dietetic Association* 26 (1950): 575–82; M. J. Franz, P. Barr, H. Holler, M. A. Powers, M. L. Wheeler, and J. Wylie-Rosett, "Exchange Lists, Revised 1985," *Journal of the American Dietetic Association* 87 (1987): 28–34; M. L. Wheeler, M. Franz, P. Barrier, H. Holler, N. Cronmiller, and L Delahanty, "Macronutrient and Kilocalorie Database for the 1995 Exchange Lists for Meal Planning: A Rationale for Clinical Practice Decisions," *Journal of the American Dietetic Association* 96 (1996): 1167–71.

3. I wore four generations of insulin pumps continuously from 1995 until November 2011, interacting with my pump twenty-four hours a day: telling it numerical stories about the sugar I planned to eat, sleeping with it, cursing at it when it didn't do what I wanted it to do. We needed to break up after one too many sequences of dysfunctional insertion sites, dermal (skin) locations on my body that had grown overused after years of catheterization.

4. Jane Dixon, "From the Imperial to the Empty Calorie: How Nutrition Relations Underpin Food Regime Transitions," *Agriculture and Human Values* 26 (2009): 323.

5. Ibid.

6. Ibid., 322.

7. Harriett Friedman, "The Political Economy of Food: A Global Crisis," *New Left Review* 197 (1993): 30–31.

8. Phillip McMichael, "A Food Regime Genealogy," *Journal of Peasant Studies* 36(1) (2009): 140.

9. John Bellamy Foster, *Marx's Ecology: Materialism and Nature* (New York: Monthly Review Press, 2000), 159–60.

10. Ibid., 158.

11. Karl Marx, *Capital,* vol. 2 (New York: Vintage Books, 1981), 949–50.

12. Geoffrey Cannon, "The Rise and Fall of Dietetics and of Nutrition Science, 4000 BCE–2000 CE," *Public Health Nutrition* 8(6A) (2005): 701–5.

13. N. Cullather, "The Foreign Policy of the Calorie," *American Historical Review* 112 (2007): 337–64; N. Fiddes, *Meat: A Natural Symbol* (London: Routledge, 1991); H. Friedmann and Phillip McMichael, "Agriculture and the State System," *Sociologica Ruralis* 39 (2) (1989): 93–97.

14. W. R. Aykroyd, *The Story of Sugar* (Chicago: Quadrangle Books, 1967), 15.

15. Sidney W. Mintz, *Sweetness and Power: The Place of Sugar in Modern History* (New York: Penguin, 1985); Herbert S. Klein, *African Slavery in Latin America and the Caribbean* (New York: Oxford University Press, 1986).

16. Hebert C. Covey and Dwight Eisnach, *What the Slaves Ate: Recollections of African American Foods and Foodways from the Slave Narratives* (Santa Barbara, Calif.: Greenwood Press, 2009).

17. Horace L. Sipple and Kristen W. McNutt, eds., *Sugars in Nutrition* (New York: Academic Press, 1974), 6; Wallace Rudell Aykroyd, *Sweet Malefactor: Sugar, Slavery, and Human Society* (London: Heinemann, 1967).

18. Food and Agricultural Organization of the United Nations, *Food Outlook: Biannual Report on Global Food Markets* (Rome: Food and Agricultural Organization of the United Nations, May 2014).

19. Rachel Schurman and William A. Munro, *Fighting for the Future of Food: Activists versus Agribusiness in the Struggle over Biotechnology* (Minneapolis: University of Minnesota Press, 2010).

20. Fred Magdoff, John Bellamy Foster, and Frederick H. Buttel, *Hungry for Profit: The Agribusiness Threat to Farmers, Food, and the Environment* (New York: Monthly Review Press, 2000).

21. Anne E. Yentsch, "Excavating the South's African American Food History," in *African American Foodways: Explorations of History and Culture,* ed. Anne L. Bower (Urbana: University of Illinois Press, 2007), 59–98.

22. Cited in Covey and Eisnach, *What the Slaves Ate,* 188.

23. W. O. Atwater and Chas D. Woods, *Dietary Studies with Reference to the Food of the Negro in Alabama in 1895 and 1896,* U.S. Department of Agriculture, Office of Experiment Stations, Bulletin No. 38 (Washington, D.C.: U.S. Government Printing Office, 1897), 19.

24. Covey and Eisnach, *What the Slaves Ate,* 213.

25. Sylvia Noble Tesh, *Hidden Arguments: Political Ideology and Disease Prevention Policy* (New Brunswick, N.J.: Rutgers University Press, 1988).

26. Delores C. S. James, "Factors Influencing Food Choices, Dietary Intake, and Nutrition-Related Attitudes among African Americans: Application of a Culturally Sensitive Model," *Ethnicity and Disease* 9(4) (2004): 351.

27. K. G. M. M. Alberti, Robert H. Eckel, Scott M. Grundy, Paul Z. Zimmet, James I. Cleeman, Karen A. Donato, Jean-Charles Fruchart, W. Philip T. James, Catherine M. Loria, and Sidney C. Smith Jr., "Harmonizing the Metabolic Syndrome: A Joint Interim Statement of the International Diabetes Federation Task Force on Epidemiology and Prevention; National Heart, Lung, and Blood Institute; American Heart Association; World Heart Federation; International Atherosclerosis Society; and International Association for the Study of Obesity," *Circulation* 1(16) (2009): 1640–45.

28. F. B. Hu, "Resolved: There Is Sufficient Scientific Evidence That Decreasing Sugar-Sweetened Beverage Consumption Will Reduce the Prevalence of Obesity and Obesity-Related Diseases," *Obesity Reviews* (14) (2013): 606–19; S. Thornley, R. Tayler, and K. Sikaris, "Sugar Restriction: The Evidence for a Drug-Free Intervention to Reduce Cardiovascular Risk," *Internal Medicine Journal* (2012): 46–58; Richard J. Johnson, Mark S. Segal, Yuri Sautin, Takahiko Nakagawa, Daniel I. Feig, Duk-Hee Kang, Michael S. Gersch, Steven Banner, and Laura G. Sanchez-Lozada, "Potential Role of Sugar (Fructose) in the Epidemic of Hypertension, Obesity, and the Metabolic Syndrome, Diabetes, Kidney Disease, and Cardiovascular Disease," *American Journal of Clinical Nutrition* 86 (2007): 899–906; Sanjay Basu, Paula Yoffe, Nancy Hills, and Robert H. Lustig, "The Relationship of Sugar to Population-Level Diabetes Prevalence: An Econometric Analysis of Repeated Cross-Sectional Data," *PLOSone* 8(2) (2013): 1–8; Roya Kelishadi, Marjan Mansourian, and Motahar Heidari-Beni, "Association of Fructose Consumption and Components of Metabolic Syndrome in Human Studies: A Systematic Review and Meta-analysis," *Nutrition* 30 (2014): 503–10; K. L. Stanhope, S. C.

Griffin, M. L. Keim, M. Ai, S. Otokozawa, K. Nakajima, E. Shaefer, and P. J. Havel, "Consumption of Fructose but Not Glucose-Sweetened Beverages Produces an Atherogenic Lipid Profile in Overweight/Obese Men and Women," *Diabetes* 56 (supplement 1, 2007): A16.

29. Luc Tappy, Kim A. Le, Christel Tran, and Nicolas Paquot, "Fructose and Metabolic Diseases: New Findings, New Questions," *Nutrition* 26 (2010): 1044–49.

30. Karim R. Saab, Jessica Kendrick, Joseph M. Yracheta, Miguel A. Lanaspa, Maisha Pollard, and Richard J. Johnson, "New Insights on the Risk for Cardiovascular Disease in African Americans: The Role of Added Sugars," *American Journal of Nephrology* 26 (2013): 247.

31. Silva Arslanian, Chittiwat Suprasongsin, and Janine E. Janosky, "Insulin Secretion and Sensitivity in Black versus White Prepubertal Health Children," *Journal of Clinical Endocrinology and Metabolism* 82(6) (1997): 1293.

32. Sushma Sharma, Lindsay Roberts, Robert H. Lustig, and Sharon E. Fleming, "Carbohydrate Intake and Cardiometabolic Risk Factors in High BMI African American Children," *Nutrition and Metabolism* 7(10) (2010): 1.

33. Q. Yang, Z. Zhang, E. W. Gregg, W. D. Flanders, R. Merritt, and F. B. Hu, "Added Sugar Intake and Cardiovascular Diseases Mortality among US Adults," *Journal of the American Medical Association Internal Medicine* 174 (2014): 516–24; F. E. Thompson, T. S. McNeel, E. C. Dowling, D. Midthune, M. Morrisette, and C. A. Zeruto, "Interrelationships of Added Sugars Intake, Socioeconomic Status, and Race/Ethnicity in Adults in the United States," *Journal of the American Dietetic Association* 109 (2009): 1376–83.

34. Carlos Novas and Nikolas Rose, "Genetic Risk and the Birth of the Somatic Individual," *Economy and Society* 29(1) (2000): 485–513.

35. Nancy Krieger and George Davey Smith, "Bodies Count and Body Counts: Social Epidemiology and Embodying Inequality," *Epidemiologic Reviews* 26 (2004): 93.

36. Marion Nestle, *Food Politics: How the Food Industry Influences Nutrition and Health* (Berkeley: University of California Press, 2002).

37. Michael K. Brown, Martin Carnoy, Elliot Currie, Troy Duster, David B. Oppenheimer, Marjorie M. Shultz, and David Wellman, *Whitewashing Race: The Myth of a Color-Blind Society* (Berkeley: University of California Press, 2003), 102; Lani Guiner and Gerald Torres, *The Miner's Canary: Enlisting Race, Resisting Power, Transforming Democracy* (Cambridge: Harvard University Press, 2002), 58.

38. Gabriel. I. Uwaifo, Tuc T. Nguyen, Margaret F. Keli, Deserea L. Russell, Jennifer C. Nicholson, Sandra H. Bonat, Jennifer R. McDuffie, and Jack Yanovski, "Differences in Insulin Secretion and Sensitivity for Caucasian and African American Prepubertal Children," *Journal of Pediatrics* 140 (2002): 673–80; B. A. Gower,

W. M. Granger, F. Franklin, R. M. Shewchuk, and M. I. Goran, "Contribution of Insulin Secretion and Clearance to Glucose-Induced Insulin Concentration in African American and Caucasian Children," *Journal of Clinical Endocrinology and Metabolism* 87 (2002): 2218–24; Chaluntorn Preeyasombat, Peter Bacchetti, Ann A. Lazar, and Robert H. Lustig, "Racial and Etiopathologic Dichotomies in Insulin Hypersecretion and Resistance in Obese Children," *Journal of Pediatrics* (2005): 474–81.

39. Gabrielle Turner-McGrievy, Deborah F. Tate, Dominic Moore, and Barry Popkin, "Taking the Bitter with the Sweet: Relationship of Supertasting and Sweet Preference with Metabolic Syndrome and Dietary Intake," *Journal of Food Science* 78(2) (2013): S336–S342; J. A. Mennella, M. Y. Pepino, and D. R. Reed, "Genetic and Environmental Determinants of Bitter Perception and Sweet Preferences," *Pediatrics* 115(2) (2005): e216–e222; M. Y. Pepino and J. A. Mennella, "Factors Contributing to Individual Differences in Sucrose Preference," *Chemical Senses* 30 (supplement 1, 2005): i319–i320; D. R. Reed and A. H. McDaniel, "The Human Sweet Tooth," *BMC Oral Health* 6 (supplement 1, 2006): S17.

40. Eugene S. Tull and Jeffrey M. Roseman, "Diabetes in African Americans," in *Diabetes in America,* 2d ed. (Bethesda, Md.: National Diabetes Data Group, 1995), 619.

41. Robyn McDermott, "Ethics, Epidemiology, and the Thrifty Gene: Biological Determinism as a Health Hazard," *Social Science and Medicine* 47(9) (1998): 1189–95.

Conclusion

1. This figure may represent an overestimate of the NIH and CDC funding levels because projects may be co-funded by different institutes within the NIH system. Additionally, some studies included in this calculation may have only a tangential relationship to metabolic syndrome.

2. Earl S. Ford, "Rarer Than a Blue Moon: The Use of a Diagnostic Code for Metabolic Syndrome in the U.S.," *Diabetes Care* 28(7) (2005): 1808–9.

3. Paul de Man, "The Resistance to Theory," *Yale French Studies 63, The Pedagogical Imperative: Teaching as a Literary Genre* (1982): 5.

4. Ivan Hannaford, *Race: The History of an Idea in the West* (Baltimore: Johns Hopkins University Press, 1996); Todd L. Savitt, *Race and Medicine in Nineteenth- and Early Twentieth-Century America* (Kent, Ohio: Kent State University Press, 2007); Harriet A. Washington, *Medical Apartheid: The Dark History of Medical Experimentation on Black Americans from Colonial Times to the Present* (New York: Doubleday, 2006).

5. Ashley Montagu, *Man's Most Dangerous Myth: The Fallacy of Race* (New York: Oxford University Press, 1994); Elazar Barkan, *The Retreat of Scientific*

Racism: Changing Concepts of Race in Britain and the United States between the World Wars (New York: Cambridge University Press, 1992); Stephen Jay Gould, *The Mismeasure of Man,* 2d ed. (New York: W. W. Norton, 1996).

6. Evelyn Nakano Glenn, *Unequal Freedom: How Race and Gender Shaped American Citizenship and Labor* (Cambridge: Harvard University Press, 2002).

7. Ash Amin, "The Remainders of Race," *Theory, Culture and Society* 27(1) (2010): 1–23; Evelyn Nakano Glenn, *Shades of Difference: Why Skin Color Matters* (Stanford, Calif.: Stanford University Press, 2009); Jennifer L. Hochschild and Vesla Weaver, "The Skin Color Paradox and the American Racial Order," *Social Forces* 86(2) (2007): 643–70; Margaret Hunter, "The Persistent Problem of Colorism: Skin Tone, Status, and Inequality," *Sociology Compass* 1 (2007): 237–54; Arun Saldanha, "Reontologising Race: The Machinic Geography of Phenotype," *Environment and Planning D: Society and Space* 24 (2006): 9–24.

8. Joseph L. Graves Jr., *The Emperor's New Clothes: Biological Theories of Race at the Millennium* (New Brunswick, N.J.: Rutgers University Press, 2001); Naomi Zack, *Philosophy of Science and Race* (London: Routledge, 2002).

9. Jinnabin Shiao, Thomas Bode, Amber Beyer, and Daniel Selvig, "The Genomic Challenge to the Social Construction of Race," *Sociological Theory* 30(2) (2012): 67–88.

10. Troy Duster, *Backdoor to Eugenics,* 2d ed. (New York: Routledge, 2003 [1990]); Anne Fausto-Sterling, "Refashioning Race: DNA and the Politics of Health Care," *Differences: A Journal of Feminist Cultural Studies* 15(3) (2004): 1–37; Lisa Gannett, "The Biological Reification of Race," *British Journal for the Philosophy of Science* 55(2) (2004): 323–45; Nancy Krieger, "Refiguring 'Race': Epidemiology, Racialized Biology, and Biological Expressions of Race Relations," *International Journal of Health Services* 30 (2000): 211–16; Dorothy A. Roberts, *Fatal Invention: How Science, Politics, and Big Business Re-create Race in the Twenty-first Century* (New York: New Press, 2011); Charis Thompson, "Race Science," *Theory, Culture and Society* 23 (2006): 547.

11. Eduardo Bonilla-Silva, *Racism without Racists: Color-Blind Racism and the Persistence of Racial Inequality in the United States* (Lanham, Md.: Roman & Littlefield, 2003); Patricia Hill Collins, *Black Sexual Politics: African Americans, Gender, and the New Racism* (New York: Routledge, 2005); Patricia J. Williams, *Seeing a Color-Blind Future: The Paradox of Race* (New York: Noonday Press, 1997); Michelle Alexander, *The New Jim Crow: Mass Incarceration in the Age of Colorblindness* (New York: New Press, 2010).

12. Collins, *Black Sexual Politics.*

13. Bonilla-Silva, *Racism without Racists.*

14. Paula S. Rothenberg, ed., *White Privilege: Essential Readings from the Other Side of Racism* (New York: Worth Publishers, 2008); Thomas Shapiro, *The Hid-*

den Costs of Being African American (New York: Oxford University Press, 2004); Williams, *Seeing a Color-Blind Future.*

15. Michael K. Brown, Martin Carnoy, Elliott Currie, Troy Duster, David B. Oppenheimer, Marjorie Schultz, and David Wellman, *Whitewashing Race: The Myth of a Color-Blind Society* (Berkeley: University of California Press, 2003).

16. Glenn, *Unequal Freedom.*

17. Bonilla-Silva, *Racism without Racists*; Brown et al., *Whitewashing Race.*

18. Brown et al., *Whitewashing Race.*

19. Lani Guinier and Gerald Torres, *The Miner's Canary: Enlisting Race, Resisting Power, Transforming Democracy* (Cambridge: Harvard University Press, 2002).

20. David Theo Goldberg, *The Racial State* (Malden, Mass.: Blackwell Publishers, 2002).

21. Bonilla-Silva, *Racism without Racists.*

22. Antonia Darder and Rodolfo D. Torres, *After Race: Racism after Multiculturalism* (New York: New York University Press, 2004); Paul Gilroy, *Against Race: Imagining Political Culture beyond the Color Line* (Cambridge: Belknap Press of Harvard University Press, 2000).

23. David Theo Goldberg, *Racist Culture: Philosophy and the Politics of Meaning* (Oxford: Blackwell Publishers, 1993).

24. James C. Scott, *Seeing like a State: How Certain Schemes to Improve the Human Condition Have Failed* (New Haven: Yale University Press, 1998).

25. See Michel Foucault, *Society Must Be Defended: Lectures at the Collège de France, 1975–1976*, ed. François Ewald, Alessandro Fontana, and Mauro Bertani, trans. David Macey (New York: Picador, 2003 [1976]).

26. Goldberg, *Racist Culture*; Howard Winant, *The World Is a Ghetto: Race and Democracy since World War II* (New York: Basic Books, 2001).

27. Derrick A. Bell, *Silent Covenants: Brown v. Board of Education and the Unfulfilled Hopes for Racial Reform* (New York: Oxford University Press, 2004); Mari J. Matsuda, Charles R. Lawrence III, Richard Delgado, and Kimberle Williams Crenshaw, *Words That Wound: Critical Race Theory, Assaultive Speech, and the First Amendment* (Boulder, Colo.: Westview Press, 1993).

28. Nadi Abu El-Haj, "The Genetic Reinscription of Race," *Annual Review of Anthropology* 36 (2007): 283–300; Sandra Soo-Jin Lee, "Biobanks of a 'Racial Kind': Mining for Difference in the New Genetics," *Patterns of Prejudice* 40(4–5) (2006): 443–60; Sara Shostak, "Environmental Justice and Genomics: Acting on the Futures of Environmental Health," *Science as Culture* 13(4) (2004): 539–62.

29. Esteban G. Burchard, Elad Ziv, Natasha Coyle, Scarlett L. Gomez, Hua Tang, Andrew J. Karter, Joanna L. Mountain, Eliseo J. Perez-Stable, Dean Sheppard, and Neil Risch, "The Importance of Race and Ethnic Background in Biomedical Reseach and Clinical Practice," *New England Journal of Medicine* 348 (2003):

1170–75; Neil Risch, Esteban Burchard, Elad Ziv, and Hua Tang, "Categorization of Humans in Biomedical Research: Genes, Race and Disease," *Genome Biology* 3(7) (2002): 1–12; Shiao et al., "The Genomic Challenge to the Social Construction of Race."

30. Lili E. Kay, *The Molecular Vision of Life: Caltech, the Rockefeller Foundation, and the Rise of the New Biology* (New York: Oxford University Press, 1993); Abby Lippman, "Prenatal Genetic Testing and Screening: Constructing Needs and Reinforcing Identities," *American Journal of Law and Medicine* 17 (1991): 15–50.

31. Richard Lewontin, "The Apportionment of Human Diversity," *Evolutionary Biology* 6 (1972): 381–98.

32. Duster, *Backdoor to Eugenics*; Sheila Jasanoff, ed., *States of Knowledge: The Co-production of Science and the Social Order* (London: Routledge, 2004).

33. Fausto-Sterling, "Refashioning Race," 1–37; Jennifer Reardon, *Race to the Finish: Identity and Governance in an Age of Genomics* (Princeton, N.J.: Princeton University Press, 2005)

34. Catherine Bliss, *Decoded: The Genomic Fight for Social Justice* (Stanford, Calif.: Stanford University Press, 2012).

35. Roberts, *Fatal Invention*, 292.

36. Osagie K. Obasogie, "Prisoners as Human Subjects: A Closer Look at the Institute of Medicine's Recommendations to Loosen Current Restrictions on Using Prisoners in Scientific Research," *Stanford Journal of Civil Rights and Civil Liberties* 6(1) (2010): 41–82; Jonathan Kahn, *Race in a Bottle: The Story of BiDil and Racialized Medicine in a Post-Genomic Age* (New York: Columbia University Press, 2012); Alondra Nelson, "Bio Science: Genetic Genealogy Testing and the Pursuit of African Ancestry," *Social Studies of Science* 38 (2008): 759–83; Anne Pollock, *Medicating Race: Heart Disease and Durable Preoccupations with Difference* (Durham, N.C.: Duke University Press, 2012); Ann Morning, *The Nature of Race: How Scientists Think and Teach about Human Difference* (Berkeley: University of California Press, 2011).

37. Janet Shim, "Constructing 'Race' across the Science–Lay Divide: Racial Formation in the Epidemiology and Experience of Cardiovascular Disease," *Social Studies of Science* 35(3) (2005): 405–36.

38. Jacqueline Stevens, "Racial Meanings and Scientific Methods: Changing Policies for NIH-Sponsored Publications Reporting Human Variation," *Journal of Health Politics, Policy and Law* 28 (2003): 1033–87; Chandra L. Ford and Collins O. Airhihenbuwa, "The Public Health Critical Race Methodology: Praxis of Antiracism Research," *Social Science and Medicine* 71 (2010): 1390–98; Camara Phyllis Jones, "'Race,' Racism, and The Practice of Epidemiology," *American Journal of Epidemiology* 154 (4) (2001): 299–304; M. Gregg Bloche, "Health Care Disparities—Science, Politics, and Race," *New England Journal of Medicine* 350 (2004): 1568–70; Brian D. Smedley, Adrienne Y. Stith, and Alan R. Nelson,

eds., *Unequal Treatment: Confronting Racial and Ethnic Disparities in Health Care* (Washington, D.C.: Committee on Understanding and Eliminating Racial and Ethnic Disparities in Health Care, Board on Health Sciences Policy, Institute of Medicine, 2003).

39. Jeremy Freese, "Genetics and the Social Science Explanation of Individual Outcomes," *American Journal of Sociology* 114 (2008): S1–35; Jeremy Freese and Sara Shostak, "Genetics and Social Inquiry," *Annual Review of Sociology* 35 (2009): 107–28; Troy Duster, "Feedback Loops in the Politics of Knowledge Production," in *The Governance of Knowledge,* ed. Nico Stehr (New Brunswick, N.J., and London: Transaction Publishers, 2004), 139–60; Hannah Landecker and Aaron Panofsky, "From Social Structure to Gene Regulation, and Back: A Critical Introduction to Environmental Epigenetics for Sociology," *Annual Review of Sociology* 39 (2013): 333–57.

ANTHONY RYAN HATCH is assistant professor in the Science in Society Program at Wesleyan University. He has held research fellowships from the American Sociological Association and the National Institute of Mental Health. His research investigates how race, gender, and power influence biomedical knowledge, technology, and practice.